Nursing and Midwifery in Ireland

About the Author

Yvonne O'Shea, RGN, RM, RNT, BA Public Administration (Health), MSc. Econ. (Policy Studies), Ph.D.

Yvonne O'Shea is the chief executive of the National Council for the Professional Development of Nursing and Midwifery in Ireland. The National Council was founded on foot of a recommendation of the *Report of the Commission on Nursing* and has led the professional development of nursing and midwifery in Ireland since 1999. During her time as chief executive, Yvonne O'Shea has been responsible for the development of a comprehensive clinical career pathway for nurses and midwives that has resulted in the creation of 1,982 clinical nurse specialist/clinical midwife specialist posts, 113 approved advanced nurse practitioner/advanced midwife practitioner posts and 66 accredited ANPs/AMPs. In addition, over 20,000 nurses and midwives have participated in additional professional development opportunities provided by the National Council to nurses and midwives in Ireland through its seminars, masterclasses and its annual conference, which attracts over 1,000 participants each year. The National Council's publications, its *Quarterly Review* and its website have become key reference points, both nationally and internationally, to monitor best practice in the professions. In addition, the National Council, in cooperation with An Bord Altranais, has been instrumental in introducing the prescribing of medications by nurses and midwives.

Yvonne O'Shea's career has included experience in general nursing, midwifery, nurse education, nurse management, nurse regulation and professional development. Prior to joining the National Council, she was chief education officer at An Bord Altranais, where her achievements included the *Review of the Scope of Practice for Nursing and Midwifery* and the introduction of the *Framework for the Scope of Nursing and Midwifery Practice.* She also spent a number of years at St James's Hospital, Dublin, first as nurse tutor and subsequently as assistant director of nursing and nurse manager in the Crest Clinical Directorate. She was the first clinical directorate nurse manager in Ireland and was nurse manager of the multidisciplinary team responsible for the successful bid to establish a new cardiac surgery unit in St James's Hospital and co-author of the successful tender document.

Nursing and Midwifery in Ireland

A Strategy for Professional Development in a Changing Health Service

Yvonne O'Shea

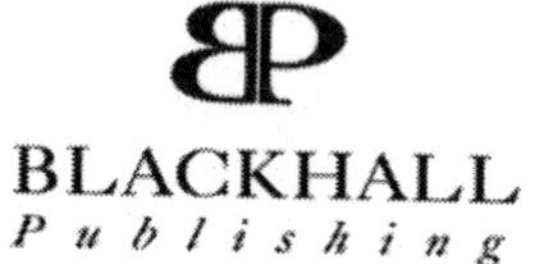

This book was typeset and published by

Blackhall Publishing
33 Carysfort Avenue
Blackrock
Co. Dublin
Ireland

e-mail: info@blackhallpublishing.com
www.blackhallpublishing.com

ISBN: 978-1-84218-161-4

A catalogue record for this book is available from the British Library.

Printed in England by Athenaeum Press Ltd.

To the Council members and staff of the National Council, and to our colleagues in the professions and in the wider Irish health services, whose support and commitment towards advancing the professional development of nursing and midwifery inspired the writing of this book.

CONTENTS

PART 2: Researching Key Stakeholders and Opinion Influencers

PART 3: The Strategic Challenges

List of Tables and Figures

List of Abbreviations

ABA	An Bord Altranais
ADON	assistant director of nursing
A&E	accident and emergency
AIDS	acquired immune deficiency syndrome
AMP	advanced midwife practitioner
ANP	advanced nurse practitioner
BNS	bachelor of nursing studies
CEO	chief executive officer
CIT	community intervention team
CME	centre of midwife education
CMHT	community mental health team
CMM	clinical midwife manager
CMS	clinical midwife specialist
CNE	centre of nurse education
CNM	clinical nurse manager
CNO	chief nursing officer
CNS	clinical nurse specialist
CPD	continuing professional development
CSO	Central Statistics Office
DATHs	Dublin academic teaching hospitals
DHSSPS	Department of Health, Social Services and Public Safety (Northern Ireland)
DoHC	Department of Health and Children
DOMINO	domiciliary care in and out of hospital
EAG	expert advisory group
ECTS	European Credit Transfer and Accumulation System
EHEA	European Higher Education Area
ENTRUST	Irish Clinical Nurse Managers Association
ERG	external reference group
ESRI	Economic and Social Research Institute
EU	European Union
EU 25	Member states of the European Union prior to the admission of Romania and Bulgaria on 1 January 2007

EU 27	Member states of the European Union following the admission of Romania and Bulgaria on 1 January 2007
EWTD	European Working Time Directive
FETAC	Further Education and Training Awards Council
FIGO	International Federation of Gynaecology and Obstetrics
GDP	gross domestic product
GFCF	gross fixed capital formation
GNI	gross national income
GP	general practitioner
HeBE	health boards executive
HIQA	Health Information and Quality Authority
HITH	hospitals in the home
HIV	human immunodeficiency virus
HR	human resources
HRB	Health Research Board
HSE	Health Service Executive
HSRP	Health Service Reform Programme
IADNAM	Irish Association of Directors of Nursing and Midwifery
ICM	International Confederation of Midwives
ICT	information and communications technology
ICU	intensive care unit
ID	intellectual disability
INO	Irish Nurses Organisation
iHIQA	Interim Health Information and Quality Authority
IR	industrial relations
LEO	Leading an Empowered Organisation programme
MBA	master of business administration
NAMIC	nursing and midwifery in the community
NCHDs	non-consultant hospital doctors
NCNM	National Council for the Professional Development of Nursing and Midwifery
NCVA	National Council for Vocational Awards
National Council	National Council for the Professional Development of Nursing and Midwifery

NEHB	North Eastern Health Board
NHO	National Hospitals' Office
NHS	National Health Service (United Kingdom)
NIDD	national intellectual disability database
NIG-EWTD	national implementation group - European Working Time Directive
NIPEC	Northern Ireland Practice and Education Council
NMPDU	nursing and midwifery planning and development unit
NSF	national service framework
NSSC	National Shared Services Centre
NTPF	National Treatment Purchase Fund
NUI Galway	National University of Ireland, Galway
NUI Maynooth	National University of Ireland, Maynooth
OECD	Organisation for Economic Co-operation and Development
OHM	Office for Health Management
PCCC	primary, community and continuing care directorate of the HSE
PCT	primary care team
PEG	percutaneous endoscopic gastronomy
PHN	public health nurse
PICC	peripheral inserted central catheter
PNA	Psychiatric Nurses Association
PRERG	post-registration nursing and midwifery education review group
RCN	registered children's nurse
RNID	registered nurse intellectual disability
RNP	registered nurse prescriber
SHA	Southern Health Area
SIPTU	Services, Industrial, Professional and Technical Union
SKILL	securing knowledge intra lifelong learning
SLMRU	skills and labour market research unit
TIGER	technology informatics guiding education reform
UCD	University College Dublin
WHO	World Health Organisation

FOREWORD

The publication of this book on the role of nursing and midwifery in the health services of the 21st century takes place almost exactly ten years after the publication of the *Report of the Commission on Nursing*. During that period, nursing and midwifery have been transformed as a result of the recommendations contained in that report. This book presents a record of the progress that has been made in those ten years, both within nursing and midwifery and in the general area of health care policy. Successive governments have made and continue to make enormous investments in the development of nursing and midwifery.

Nurses and midwives have always been at the heart of healthcare delivery in Ireland. They are in the frontline of service delivery and advocate on behalf of patients and clients within the services. Yvonne O'Shea offers us an account of the role in the health services past and present. She reflects on how the future development of the health services will require a transformation of the culture of nursing and midwifery professions with a greater emphasis on collaborative working.

The development of healthcare in Ireland relies on the existence of a strong cohort of professional nursing and midwifery expertise, capable of spanning institutional boundaries reaching into the communities where the patients and clients of the services live. This book provides an insight into how the continued development of the professions can be empowered in a manner that is responsive to the needs of the services.

Mary Harney, TD
Minister for Health and Children

FOREWORD

Nurses and midwives have a unique role to play in managing and strengthening the relationship between patients and clients and the health service. They provide practical help and advice, reassurance, comfort and support. They also empower patients, clients and their families to take ownership of many aspects of their own health care. This is at the heart of the *essence of nursing*.

The importance and potential of nursing and midwifery in the delivery of modern health services is immense. Recent legislation and education to provide for medicine prescribing by nurses and midwives is the most recent example of change which is unlocking this potential. Hopefully it will pave the way for more empowering changes.

This and many other examples are highlighted in this book as it celebrates the richness of the role that nursing and midwifery can play in the health services of the future.

It is a very timely and welcome contribution to the current health transformation programme. It provides a strategic analysis of the role of nursing and midwifery and presents challenges to all of us who have an interest in strengthening the profession.

It asks what nursing and midwifery professionals can do to contribute to shaping and building a modern health service that is capable of consistently responding to the community's evolving needs within the resources available. It also promotes the importance of sound, evidence-based knowledge as the cornerstone of professional competence.

Importantly, the book presents a vision of the profession as an essential bridge linking acute and community-based care settings and urges the integration of the services to make access and the journey for patients easier and more convenient. This is an integrated approach, which the HSE fully supports.

Professor Brendan Drumm
Chief Executive
Health Service Executive

INTRODUCTION

The quality of any health care system throughout the world is, to a great extent, determined by the level of commitment it makes to nursing and midwifery care and to those who practice as nurses and midwives. There is no doubt that nursing and midwifery are changing and having to adapt to the many influences which affect them today, especially the cultural, economic, technological and political factors.

Whatever the changes, there will always be a variety of roles for nurses and midwives, the key one being the delivery of up-to-date, evidence-based, sensitive health care. In order to do this efficiently and effectively in the world today, especially in Ireland, nurses and midwives need to understand where they are coming from, the context of health care today and the future direction in which they are heading.

This book by Yvonne O'Shea reviews the past, the present and the prospects for the future. It is an excellent overview of the subject, of where the role of nursing and midwifery stands and of where many local nursing and midwifery leaders and other key players in the health services in Ireland feel it is heading. I was privileged to have been the external examiner for the research work on which this book is based, and therefore have seen at close hand what has been achieved.

This has been a significant major review carried out by a determined highly professional nurse who is strongly committed to nursing and midwifery in Ireland. Yvonne O'Shea has done a tremendous job in not only achieving the aims of her research, but in writing and publishing a book (so soon after her research), which I am sure will become a classic historical reference for the future.

Nursing and health care in Ireland should be proud that it has such a talented nurse who is prepared not only to proactively go and find out what is happening to her profession, but is also keen to help implement a strategic direction for nursing and midwifery over the next ten years.

I strongly recommend this book to all seriously minded and committed nurses and midwives and hope that it will be used as a catalyst and motivator for discussion and future directions in nursing and midwifery not only in Ireland but in health care decisions around the world.

Professor Sir George Castledine
Professor and International Consultant in Nursing Care
The Institute of Ageing and Health
Birmingham
UK

Preface

Over the past ten years, nursing and midwifery in Ireland have experienced a considerable number of changes, which were driven principally by the *Report of the Commission on Nursing*, published in 1998,[1] and the Health Service Reform Programme,[2] announced in 2003. In the same period, Irish society has become wealthier and more culturally diverse, creating new challenges for nursing and midwifery. This book sets out to identify the role for nursing and midwifery in the health services of the future in Ireland and to formulate a strategy for the professional development of nursing and midwifery that will prepare them to fulfil that role.

The book has three parts. Part 1 establishes the context within which the professions of nursing and midwifery operate in Ireland, and traces the evolution and development of the professions. It also provides an analysis of the key policy developments that have taken place in recent years and their implications for nursing and midwifery. The impact of the *Report of the Commission on Nursing* on the professions is reviewed with a particular emphasis on the work of the National Council for the Professional Development of Nursing and Midwifery, and the way in which the role of nurses and midwives has developed in recent years. It also examines the question of leadership and empowerment in nursing and midwifery, both of which are key factors in the development of the professions.

Part 2 is based on a set of seventy-seven semi-structured interviews with senior figures in the health services, such as policymakers, service managers, medical consultants, educators and leaders of nursing and midwifery, as well as group interviews with senior nurse managers and educators.

Part 3 draws on the findings from the research and formulates a strategy for the professional development of nursing and midwifery. The strategy is based on an examination of the strengths, weaknesses, opportunities and threats facing the professions. A statement of vision reflects what nursing and midwifery are likely to look and feel like in the health services of the future in Ireland. A mission statement, which encompasses the core elements of the essence of nursing, outlines the central role and purpose of nursing and midwifery in line with the needs of the service. The overarching strategy outlines what the long-term objectives of the professions should be in order to meet the expectations of the major stakeholders. A number of key strategies are identified aimed at achieving these objectives. The strategy concludes with an analysis of the strategic action programmes and measures of success that would need to be implemented, while at the same time identifying the key stakeholders that would be involved in the implementation process. The book closes with a summary of the next key steps required, including the need to debate and adopt the strategy at national level and set time-based review points.

Nursing and Midwifery in Ireland: A Strategy for Professional Development in a Changing Health Service is published at a time of significant change within the health services in Ireland. It is intended as a contribution to ensuring that nursing and midwifery take their place at the heart of health service transformation, in partnership with other key players, for the benefit of the patients and clients of the services.

I would like to acknowledge the following, without whose contribution and support this book would not have been possible: participants in the interviews and focus groups, for their cooperation and invaluable input; Professor Cecily Begley, Faculty of Health Sciences, School of Nursing and Midwifery, University of Dublin, Trinity College, for her supervision and guidance in preparing my thesis on this subject submitted in fulfilment of the requirements for the degree of Doctor in Philosophy (Ph.D.) (Nursing and Midwifery); and my family and friends.

Their suggestions, comments and advice have shaped the development of this book from dissertation to publication, but responsibility for any omissions or errors lies with me alone.

Yvonne O'Shea

PART 1

A Time of Change for the Professions

CHAPTER 1

The Essence of Nursing

Florence Nightingale, in her classic *Notes on Nursing: What it Is and What it is Not*,[3] speaks of nursing as aiding the reparative process of nature through the proper use of fresh air, light, warmth, cleanliness, quiet and the proper selection and administration of diet. She describes nursing as the care that puts the patient in the best possible condition for nature to act. She also speaks of taking charge, that is, not just doing what is necessary oneself, but making sure that everyone else does so too. An essential feature of nursing is what she terms 'sound and ready observation'. This is a cumulative process that focuses on all parts of the body, cognisant of the fact that frequently the patients cannot speak for themselves. Nightingale refers to this as 'the faculty of observation'. Sound and ready observation is, according to Nightingale, essential in a nurse. Thus it is through controlling the environment, providing a wide range of personal services, careful observation and taking charge that the nurse, according to Nightingale, aids the reparative process of nature.

Nightingale's view of nursing is still present in much of modern literature on the role of nurses and midwives, although the emphasis has shifted away from control of the environment to interaction with the individual. This reflects the fact that, in modern institutional settings, the nurse or midwife is less in control of the environment. In recent times, perhaps the most widely used definition of nursing is the one proposed by Virginia Henderson.[4] According to Henderson, the unique function of the nurse is to assist individuals, sick or well, in the performance of those activities contributing to health or its recovery (or to peaceful death) that they would perform unaided if they had the necessary strength, will or knowledge and to do this in such a way as to help them regain independence as soon as possible.

In 1995, a World Health Organisation (WHO) expert committee on nursing practice[5] considered Henderson's definition of nursing and concluded that, while the definition provides a sound foundation for describing nursing as it relates to individuals in a wide range of health care situations, it does not take account of issues arising from the changing orientations of health systems and policies or from the new roles and responsibilities that have evolved for nursing personnel. Nursing roles have changed in response to many factors, including technological advances, the transfer of tasks from medicine to nursing, the expansion of health care coverage through community nursing, the absence of physicians in some areas and the reorientation of health care systems to primary care. In response to these changes, the committee proposed the following three-part, functional description of nursing:

1. Nursing helps individuals, families and groups to determine and achieve their physical, mental and social potential, and to do so within the challenging context of the environment in which they live and work. The nurse requires competence to develop and perform functions that promote and maintain health as well as prevent ill health. Nursing also includes the planning and giving of care during illness and rehabilitation, and encompasses the physical, mental and social aspects of life as they affect health, illness, disability and dying.
2. Nursing promotes the active involvement of the individual and his or her family, friends, social group and community as appropriate, in all aspects of health care, thus encouraging self-reliance and self-determination while promoting a healthy environment.
3. Nursing is both an art and a science. It requires the understanding and application of specific knowledge and skills and it draws on knowledge and techniques derived from the humanities and the physical, social, medical and biological sciences.

The value of this contribution from the WHO is that it provides a comprehensive description of the work of a nurse. It is a modern day adaptation of the Nightingale view of the nurse and incorporates Henderson's focus on the individual. It also emphasises the role of the nurse as an educator (of individuals and families), as a promoter of health, and the importance of knowledge and skills, science and expertise.

Other writers have provided deep insights into the philosophy and value system that underpin the role of the nurse. In 1999, Kitson[6] identified what she described as the first essence or essential element in nursing: the philosophical and moral recognition of nursing as a person-centred activity. This is based on an acknowledgement of the uniqueness of the individual and the need for a set of attitudes and behaviours for the nurse to operate in a person-centred way.

These include paying attention to detail; uncovering meaning in everyday situations; being attentive and available, reliable and true to promises; and understanding the importance of each person's own biography and how he or she is seeking to gain an understanding of what is happening to him or her.

Other commentators and theorists[7] have used a variety of approaches to explain how nurses can provide patient-centred care. These include the development of 'mutuality', or a demonstration of the nurse's ability to hold an unconditional positive regard for the other person.[8] It also includes being able to focus in on significant events, conditions or situations that enable the nurse to help each person feel intact.[9] Benner[10] elaborates on the powers of observation of the nurse and how these develop over time and experience to enable the 'expert' nurse to exercise 'clinical judgement' based on his or her experience and observations and to develop 'clinical wisdom'. It is part of the nurse's reflective practice. This, according to Kitson, is part of a nurse's sensing and intuitive role, part of the shared experience between the nurse and the human being that requires nursing, each one sharing the experience, each one recognising the contribution of the other. It is this philosophy, says Kitson, with which nursing should start and finish.

This complements, but perhaps goes further than, Nightingale's emphasis on 'sound and ready observation' as being essential in a nurse. Nightingale's emphasis was on observation of the physical environment and the physical well-being of the patient. In this case, it extends to the whole person and the human circumstances in the environment. It includes an element of relationship building as an essential requirement for the nurse to be able to contribute to an individual's ability to 'feel intact'.

In addition to this, however, Kitson says that nursing also requires a set of practical skills that constitute the essential elements that make up patient-centred care. These include:

1. **Essential care**: This includes putting the patient in the right environment to ensure optimal recovery. This is similar to Nightingale's emphasis on controlling the environment. It is perhaps the most important basic job of the nurse. It provides an answer to the key question, how can I ensure that the immediate environment is conducive to optimal care?
2. **Technological care**: This includes monitoring and observation skills, similar to Nightingale's 'sound and ready observation' and Benner's 'reflective practice' of the expert nurse as the basis for sound clinical judgement that require an understanding of pathology, treatments, side-effects and potential hazards. This provides an answer to the question, how stable and predictable are the patient's physiological functions?
3. **Psychosocial/emotional care/information and education**: This includes interpersonal skills such as the ability to communicate, inform and educate patients, relatives and their carers. This provides an answer to the question: how stable and predictable are the patient's psychosocial and emotional states? It also provides an answer to the question, what does the patient need to know and learn about his or her condition or situation?
4. **Continuity and coordination**: This includes knowing how to provide a continuous, uninterrupted package of care, coordinated across geographic and service boundaries as well as between members of the health care team and the patient's own family (similar to what Nightingale referred to as 'taking charge'). This provides an answer to the question, how can I ensure that the patient experiences care that is uninterrupted and coordinated?

There are a number of common elements that run through these definitions and interpretations of nursing. Together, they make up what can be described as the essence of nursing, the core elements of which are:

1. **Person-centred care**: The individual experiences care in such a way as to feel that the nurse or midwife acts at all times in the interests of the person involved.
2. **Relationship-based care**: The experience of person-centred care is based on a relationship of empathy and of connection. The relationship is based on respect and consideration for the individual. It is animated by the values of equality, esteem, meaning, safety and trust.
3. **Holistic care**: The care provided by the nurse and midwife focuses on the totality of the person – physical, psychosocial and emotional. It is also sensitive to the cultural circumstances of the individual and is based on the value of respect for diversity.
4. **Education and promotion**: The care provided by the nurse or midwife is focused on promoting self-reliance and independence in individuals. This includes providing them with the wherewithal to be able to become independent. It extends beyond the individuals to their families and communities in order to ensure that support mechanisms are empowered to assist.
5. **Coordination**: Nurses and midwives ensure that individuals have access to whatever is required to assist them to achieve self-reliance and independence. This includes coordinating the inputs of other professionals, making technology available as required and taking charge of environmental management issues that affect the well-being of the individual.
6. **Knowledge-based care**: Nurses and midwives invest in their own education and development, fully aware that clinical wisdom comes about as a result of experience combined with knowledge and understanding. Competence development is an essential ingredient in the accountability values that nurses and midwives build into their professional practice. Nurses and midwives see themselves as professionals who combine science and art in the interests of individuals under their care.

A number of nursing theorists have sought to articulate this essence of nursing in the form of 'nursing models'. These models have served as a framework for developing the theory and practice of nursing.

The Neuman model of nursing[11] is a conceptual framework, or a visual representation, for thinking about humans and nurses and their interactions. This model views the person as a layered, multidimensional whole who is in constant dynamic interaction with the environment. The layers represent various levels of defence protecting the core being. The two major components in the model are stress reactions and systemic feedback loops. The patient/client reacts to stress with lines of defence and resistance. Continuous feedback loops fine-tune the lines of defence and resistance so as to achieve a maximal level of stability. The patient/client is in continuous and dynamic interaction with the environment. The exchanges between the environment and the patient/client are reciprocal, each one being influenced by the other. The goal is to achieve optimal system stability and balance. Prevention is the main nursing intervention to achieve this balance. Primary, secondary and tertiary prevention activities are used to attain, retain and maintain system balance.[12]

Patricia Benner takes the Dreyfus model of skill acquisition and applies it to nursing.[13] According to this model, nurses progress from being novices to experts principally though the knowledge they gain in the practice of nursing. In other words, the knowledge embodied in the practical world is important for the development of the nurse's skills and ability to care. Her area of concern is not how to do nursing but rather, 'how do nurses learn to do nursing?'

The Orem model of nursing was developed in 1985 by Dorothea Orem[14] and is also known as the 'self-care' model of nursing. It is used, in particular, in rehabilitation and primary care settings where the patient is encouraged to be as independent as possible. The Orem model is based upon the philosophy that all 'patients wish to care for themselves'. Self-care requisites are groups of needs or requirements that Orem identified. They are classified as either universal self-care requisites (those needs that all people have), developmental self-care requisites (those needs that relate to development of the individual) or health deviation requisites (those needs that arise as a result of a patient's condition). When individuals are unable to meet their own self-care requisites, a self-care deficit occurs. It is the job of the registered nurse to determine these deficits, and define a support modality based on an analysis of the dependency level of the individual. The support modality will be designed to provide either total compensation or partial compensation, or as an educative and supportive intervention.

The Roper, Logan and Tierney[15] model of nursing is a model of care based upon activities of living. The model is based loosely upon the activities of living evolved from the work of Virginia Henderson in 1966.[16] Whereas Henderson identified fourteen activities in which people engage in order to live, Roper et al. use twelve. These are:

1. Maintaining a safe environment
2. Communication
3. Breathing
4. Eating and drinking
5. Elimination
6. Washing and dressing
7. Thermoregulation
8. Mobilisation
9. Working and playing
10. Expressing sexuality
11. Sleeping
12. Death and dying.

These activities should be considered within the dependence–independence continuum. They are used to guide the initial assessment of a patient upon admission, and are referred to again as the patient's condition is reviewed and the care plan revised. To provide effective care, all the patient's needs (which are identified by investigating the patient's specific requirements relative to each activity) must be met as practicably as possible. The model also incorporates a life-span continuum, where the individual passes from full dependence at birth, to full independence in the midlife, and returns to full dependence in old age or death.

Considered together, these models of nursing reveal the essence of nursing activity, namely appropriate and responsive care of the patient's needs, and from that activity the identity of nursing may be deduced. They translate the essence of nursing into frameworks for theory and practice. They also serve to distinguish clearly the nursing model of care from the medical model.

The term 'medical model' was coined by the psychiatrist R.D. Laing[17] and denotes the set of processes and procedures in which all doctors are trained. This set includes complaint identification, history-taking, physical examination, ancillary tests if needed, diagnosis, treatment, and prognosis with or without treatment. The medical model aims to find medical treatments for diagnosed symptoms and syndromes and treats the human body as a very complex mechanism. It drives research and theorising about physical or psychological difficulties on the basis of causation and remediation. In this, it is quite distinct from the holistic approach of the nursing model, based on care for the needs of the individual and the development of a relationship within which this care is provided.

As nursing and midwifery move into areas of specialisation and advanced practice, it is important that the essence of nursing and midwifery is promoted and maintained. In Ireland, the National Council for the Professional Development of Nursing and Midwifery (National Council) requires all those who wish to be recognised as clinical nurse specialists/clinical midwife specialists (CNSs/CMSs) or advanced nurse practitioners/ advanced midwife practitioners (ANPs/AMPs) to demonstrate the contribution their work makes to nursing and midwifery practice. Thus, where the specialist or advanced practice is to be conducted in a particular area of clinical practice, what is required is a demonstration of the nursing and midwifery contribution to the area of practice.[18]

In developing areas of specialisation and advanced practice for nurses and midwives, therefore, it is important that the medical model does not dominate. It is equally important that an economic model of organisational and structural change within the health services does not dominate. Thus, for example, in developing the role of the nurse and midwife in the community, it is important that it is not driven solely by the need to achieve efficiencies or to substitute for the role of the general practitioner (GP) or other health care professionals. Nurses and midwives have an important part to play in adapting to the demands of efficiency and organisational change, but must do so while remaining true to their own professional identity. It is only in this way that the professions of nursing and midwifery can make their own specific contribution to the health of individuals and their families in society.

At times of change it is important to have a touchstone that ensures that core values and ideals are not lost in the maelstrom of evolution and change. This is particularly important in nursing and midwifery in Ireland today, as it faces up to a future that holds many challenges, such as adaptation to new ways of working, new organisational structures, new relationships with other professionals, and new social and cultural changes. A strategy for the professional development of nursing and midwifery in a changing Irish health service must be imbued with the values and ideals that are at the heart of the professions – the essence of nursing and midwifery. They inform the identity of the professions and will be a central component of the strategy that emerges.

CHAPTER 2

Nursing and Midwifery in Ireland

The development of a statute-based system of self-regulation that requires nurses and midwives to be eligible for inclusion on a register is at the base of the professionalism of nursing and midwifery. This professionalism has evolved over the years in response to service and professional developments, culminating most recently in a radical review of the roles of nursing and midwifery by the Commission on Nursing. The findings and recommendations of the Commission had profound implications for the development of the professions and for the role of nurses and midwives in the health services. It has resulted in the introduction of a number of significant changes in the professions, in particular the introduction of a clinical career pathway developed by the National Council.

Developments in the ten years since the Commission completed its work have included the emergence of an increased number of nurse-/midwife-led services, the involvement of nurses and midwives in prescribing, and major changes in the demands being placed on nurse and midwife managers. There has also been a radical transformation in the provision of educational opportunities for nurses and midwives, at both pre- and post-registration levels, including increased professional development opportunities. Recent developments have also included an increased emphasis on the creation of joint appointments between clinical and educational settings.

Divisions of the Register

There are a number of divisions of the Register of Nurses maintained by An Bord Altranais (ABA). The principal divisions and the number of individuals registered in each at the end of

2006 were:

- General Nursing (69,725)
- Midwifery (17,275)
- Psychiatric Nursing (12,043)
- Intellectual Disability Nursing (4,609)
- Children's Nursing (4,844)
- Public Health Nursing (2,797).[19]

General Nursing

At a single stroke the *Nurses Registration Act, 1919*[20] provided nursing and midwifery with their statutory basis and established a Register of general nurses. The Nurses Acts of 1950, 1961, and 1985[21] retained this register and formalised the authority under which general nurses could practise.[22] At present, over 55,000 nurses on the live register have general nursing qualifications.[23]

General nurse training has seen much development and increasing academic recognition. The introduction of the four-year degree programme for the pre-registration education of nurses in 2002, on foot of a recommendation by the Commission on Nursing, was the first time that officialdom put in place the conditions for making nursing education visible and, indirectly, recognising the contribution that nursing could make to health care.[24]

Midwifery

The accepted international definition of the midwife in Ireland is the one that has been adopted by the International Confederation of Midwives (ICM), the International Federation of Gynaecology and Obstetrics (FIGO) and the WHO.[25] This definition, which is endorsed by An Bord Altranais,[26] states:

> A midwife is a person who, having been regularly admitted to a midwifery educational programme, duly recognised in the country in which it is located, has successfully completed the prescribed course of studies in midwifery and has acquired the requisite qualifications to be registered and/or legally licensed to practise midwifery.
>
> She must be able to give the necessary supervision, care and advice to women during pregnancy, labour and the postpartum period, to conduct deliveries on her own responsibility and to care for the newborn and the infant. This care includes preventative measures,

the detection of abnormal conditions in mother and child, the procurement of medical assistance and the execution of emergency measures in the absence of medical help. She has an important task in health counselling and education, not only for the women, but also within the family and the community. The work should involve antenatal education and preparation for parenthood and extends to certain areas of gynaecology, family planning and child care. She may practise in hospitals, clinics, health units, domiciliary conditions or in any other service.

The *Report of the Commission on Nursing* identified the midwifery profession as being distinct from nursing, and as possessing exclusive skills in relation to maternity care. Nevertheless, many midwives feel confined by obstetric practitioners. Midwifery-led care has long been an aspiration of midwives and women in Ireland.[27] The *Report of the Maternity Review Group* in the former North Eastern Health Board (NEHB) proposed the setting up of two midwife-led units attached to conventional maternity units in the NEHB.[28] Two such units were opened in July 2004 and are currently being evaluated. Many midwives have stated that they are now actively seeking opportunities to practise midwifery within settings that provide midwives with autonomy and pregnant women with alternative choices in childbirth.[29] There are examples of innovative community practice taking place at present, such as the service provided by the Southern Health Area (SHA), which employs independent midwives to provide domiciliary maternity services. The evaluation of the pilot scheme DOMINO (domiciliary care in and out of hospital) in the National Maternity Hospital showed that it was extremely successful and viable and, given sufficient funding, was sustainable in the long term.[30] The evaluation made a strong case for the development of similar schemes in other Dublin maternity hospitals and in maternity units around the country.

Until recently, the only pathway to becoming a midwife was to undertake general nursing, followed by a two-year post-registration diploma programme. A direct entry degree programme in midwifery commenced in September 2006.

Psychiatric Nursing

The publication of the policy report *The Psychiatric Services: Planning for the Future*[31] by the Department of Health in 1984 set out the blueprint for a community mental health service in Ireland. It outlined major changes in the mental health services, notably moving the delivery of in-patient services from large psychiatric hospitals to units in general hospitals. There was a greater emphasis on rehabilitating the mentally ill and relocating services into mainstream medical care and especially into the community. This shift in policy represented a major change in the role of psychiatric nurses and provided a unique opportunity for development of skills and roles.[32] The publication in 2006 of the most recent policy review for psychiatric services, *A Vision for Change: Report of the Expert Group on Mental Health Policy*,[33] re-emphasised the importance of the community-based dimension of psychiatric care through the promotion of the concept of community mental health teams (CMHTs), consisting of different health care professionals providing services within their catchment area.

In 1994, a diploma in nursing programme was set up in the former Western Health Board, in conjunction with the National University of Ireland, Galway (NUI Galway), and was extended to all schools of nursing, including psychiatry, in the following four years. In 2002, along with general and 'mental handicap' nursing, the first pre-registration degree programme commenced in psychiatric nursing.

Intellectual Disability Nursing

The registered intellectual disability nurse provides a range of services across a wide variety of locations, addressing the particular and complex needs of clients, and requiring particular skills and personal qualities distinct from those in other disciplines of nursing.

The first training schools offering a three-year course in mental handicap nursing opened in 1959. Mental handicap nursing in the early 1960s focused on the treatment and care of the severely disabled of all ages, and the treatment, care and training of the lower ranges of moderately disabled children and moderately and mildly disabled adults and of others with mental handicaps.[34] More schools of mental handicap nursing were established from that time until 2002, and the syllabus of training has been revised on several occasions to reflect trends in care and service provision.[35] The *Nurses Rules, 2004*[36] replaced the title 'registered mental handicap nurse' with the title 'registered nurse intellectual disability' (RNID).

Children's Nursing

Specialist hospitals for the care of sick infants and children have been a feature of the health service in Ireland for close on two centuries. The National Children's Hospital in Harcourt Street, Dublin, was founded in 1821, and this was followed by the founding of the Children's Hospital, Temple Street, Dublin, in 1872. A third children's hospital, Our Lady's Hospital for Sick Children in Crumlin, Dublin, was founded in 1956.[37] The first school of paediatric nurse education was established in the Temple Street Hospital in 1883.

As with the pre-registration programmes pertaining to the other branches of nursing, there have been changes to the paediatric programme, culminating in the present system. The one-year post-registration programme is a higher diploma or postgraduate diploma. Many paediatric nurses currently working in centres outside Dublin are required to hold an additional registerable qualification, usually in general nursing. The *Nurses Rules, 2004* replaced the title 'registered sick children's nurse' with 'registered children's nurse' (RCN).

Public Health Nursing

Public health has been described as organised social and political effort and health promotion for the benefit of populations, families and individuals.[38] There are 2,797 public health nurses (PHNs) on the active Register, making them the largest group of professionals working in the community.[39] PHNs practise as part of a multidisciplinary team to deliver domiciliary care and have a wide remit, encompassing primary, secondary and tertiary care at three levels: individual, family and community.[40] They have responsibility for providing a nursing service in the community to multiple client groups with any type of condition, and public health nursing is an amalgamation of services incorporating midwifery, public health and home nursing.[41] Their role is threefold, combining that of manager, clinician and health promoter.[42]

The wide range of abilities and responsibilities of a PHN is reflected in the educational and experiential preparation required to register as one. Formerly, this took a minimum of eight years, as the PHN until recently had to be registered as a general nurse and as a registered midwife, had to have obtained a higher diploma in public health nursing and, in addition, have a minimum of two years experience in clinical practice.[43] Under the *Nurses Rules, 2004* nurses registered in divisions other than general nursing are eligible to apply for public health nursing courses, the requirement for a midwifery qualification has been removed and a module in maternity and child health has been substituted, reducing the preparation time to five years.[44]

The Commission on Nursing

The *Report of the Commission on Nursing*, published in 1998, represented the most comprehensive review of nursing and midwifery ever conducted in Ireland. The Commission on Nursing was established following a period of considerable industrial unrest among nurses and midwives about the conditions under which they were employed, the career development options open to them, the nature and range of educational services available and the general perception of the professions. In 1997, nurses and midwives voted for strike action. The setting up of the Commission on Nursing by the Government, following a recommendation from the Labour Court, averted a strike.[45]

The agreed terms of reference were as follows:

'The Commission will examine and report on the role of nurses in the health services including:

- 'The evolving role of nurses, reflecting their professional development and their role in the overall management of services
- 'Promotional opportunities and related difficulties
- 'Structural and work changes appropriate for the effective and efficient discharge of that role
- 'The requirements placed on nurses, both in training and the delivery of services
- 'Segmentation of the grade
- 'Training and educational requirements.'

The original terms of reference also stated that, in its recommendations, the Commission should seek 'to provide a secure basis for the further development of nursing in the context of anticipated changes in health services, their organisation and delivery.' In light of discussions during the Commission's consultation process, and following agreement by An Bord Altranais, the Commission sought and secured an extension of its terms of reference to include 'the role and function of An Bord Altranais generally, including, inter alia, education and professional development, regulation and protection of the citizen.'[46]

One of the recommendations of the Commission on Nursing was that a monitoring committee would be established which would issue yearly reports. (This Committee was established and held its first meeting on 1 February 2000.) It was envisaged that recommendations without a suggested timescale would be implemented as soon as practicable and, in any event, by the end of 2002. The Commission, in addition to timescales given in its report, identified four recommendations as urgent. These were:

1. The establishment of the nursing education forum (for pre-registration education)
2. The establishment of the National Council (for post-registration education)
3. The establishment of the nursing and midwifery planning and development units (NMPDUs) in each health board, all of which should be established at the earliest possible date
4. The introduction of legislation amending the *Nurses Act, 1985*,[47] which should be introduced before the Oireachtas by early 1999.

When the report was published, the then Minister for Health and Children, Mr Brian Cowen, TD,[48] referred to the vacuum that had existed in providing direction to the professions of nursing and midwifery and spoke of the impact that the report would have on freeing the professions from controls, practices and attitudes that have held nursing back and prevented it from achieving its full potential in the health services and in society. The Commission's report provided a comprehensive framework, or blueprint, for the development of the professions into the future. This included the creation of a number of new bodies with responsibility for the development of the professions such as the nursing policy division in the Department of Health and Children, the NMPDUs and the National Council.

Two of the most far-reaching recommendations of the *Report of the Commission on Nursing* were the introduction of a pre-registration degree programme for nurses and midwives superseding/succeeding the certificate and diploma programmes as the qualifying programme for entry to the professions, and the determination of a comprehensive clinical career pathway, from generalist nurse to clinical nurse specialist (CNS) and to advanced nurse practitioner (ANP). There was an equivalent career pathway for midwives, from generalist midwife to clinical midwife specialist (CMS) to advanced midwife practitioner (AMP). The report introduced for the first time in Ireland the concept of CNS/CMS and ANP/AMP as part of the clinical career pathway for nurses and midwives. The implementation of these recommendations has transformed the professions in recent years and promises to provide a platform for the further development of the contribution of the professions to the health services of the future (see Appendix 5).

Role of the National Council

The National Council for the Professional Development of Nursing and Midwifery was established as an independent statutory agency[49] with responsibility for the development of a clinical career pathway for nurses and midwives. It is responsible for determining the appropriate level of qualification and experience necessary for entry into specialist practice and advanced practice for nursing and midwifery. In addition, the National Council provides a range of professional development and support services appropriate to each step on the clinical career pathway. These include the provision of funding to support additional continuing educational initiatives for nurses and midwives in cooperation with the NMPDUs. The National Council also works closely with the NMPDUs on a wide range of strategic development issues, which include the development of clinical specialist and advanced practitioner posts and the promotion of research in nursing and midwifery.

The National Council has taken the lead in the introduction of important policy initiatives, such as the involvement of nurses and midwives in prescribing medicinal preparations (in partnership with An Bord Altranais), the promotion of research in nursing and midwifery (in partnership with the Health Research Board), and the promotion of educational programmes to support the clinical career pathway (in partnership with third-level institutions and the centres of nurse and midwife education). The National Council also provides masterclasses and seminars on nursing and midwifery topics, organises an annual conference on professional development issues, and provides an interactive portal website that acts as host for a wide range of nursing and midwifery specialist interest groups. The National Council offers extensive professional advice at individual and organisational levels (see Appendix 6).

Development of the Clinical Career Pathway

Until 1998 there was no framework for developing a clinical career pathway in Ireland, although there were some initiatives at a local level aimed at developing specialists in nursing. Thus, for example, in 1996 the first nurse acknowledged to be practising at an advanced level in Ireland was appointed on a pilot basis in an emergency department in a Dublin hospital and was known as an emergency nurse practitioner. Also in 1996, a *Tender for Establishment and Provision of Cardiac Surgery Services at St. James's Hospital* in Dublin contained a proposal to include four nurse practitioner posts as part of the staffing complement.[50] The roots of specialism in nursing and midwifery in Ireland can be found in the *Report of the Working Party on General Nursing*,[51] which recommended the appointment of specialist nurses to enhance nursing care by providing specialist nursing advice to other nurses. It was the *Report of the Commission on Nursing* that recommended the establishment of a comprehensive clinical career pathway framework to encourage experienced nurses and midwives to remain in clinical practice and use their expert skills to improve patient outcomes and respond to health policy developments. The clinical career pathway leads from generalist to specialist to advanced practice. Levels on the pathway are linked with levels of educational preparation, responsibility and autonomy, and to different points on a pay scale that reflect these different levels of responsibility. Responsibility for monitoring the development of the clinical career pathway framework and for monitoring its development was assigned to the National Council.

By July 2008, such has been the level of acceptance that there were 1,982 approved CNS/CMS posts, 113 approved ANP/AMP posts and 66 accredited ANPs/AMPs. Appendices 1 and 2 contain lists of approved ANP/AMP and CNS/CMS posts, respectively, that had been approved by July 2008.[52]

The clinical career pathway is designed to ensure that nurses and midwives can fulfil their professional role within a range of care settings and working at different grades and with different levels of clinical autonomy. These grades include those of the generalist nurse at staff nurse and staff midwife grade, the specialist nurse/midwife at CNS/CMS grade and the advanced practice nurse/midwife at ANP/AMP grade.[53] The respective roles of staff nurses, staff midwives, CNSs, CMSs, ANPs and AMPs are distinguished by their scope of practice, educational preparation and levels of clinical decision-making, responsibility and autonomy.

Current Career Pathways

Table 1 provides a general reference grid for current career pathways in nursing and midwifery, based on the recommendations contained in the *Report of the Commission on Nursing*.

Direct entry to all of the branches of nursing and to midwifery is now available to those seeking to become nurses or midwives. The basic qualification for both professions is now a degree, which qualifies the individual to be registered as a nurse or midwife on the Register. Career path progression is then divided into three general areas: clinical practice, education and management. Clinical career options are divided between acute, primary and specialised services. Career options in education are divided between the third-level sector and the centres for nurse and midwife education (CNEs/CMEs). The management career pathway reflects the recommendations of the Commission for a clearer definition of the various levels of management provided for nursing and midwifery. The Commission recommended that there should not be a separate pathway for research, asserting that research should be integrated into the clinical and academic career pathways. Finally, a report was prepared for the Commission on the question of joint appointments between clinical and academic institutions in nursing and midwifery.

Table 1: Current Career Pathways in Nursing and Midwifery

Branch/ division of the Register	General nursing	Midwifery (since 2006)	Psychiatric nursing	Intellectual disability nursing	Children's nursing (integrated with general nursing since 2006)
Entry qualification	Degree				
Role	Registered staff nurse/midwife				
Role progression	**Clinical (hospital and community)**		**Educational**		**Management (hospital and community)**
Acute services	Registered staff nurse/midwife Clinical nurse/midwife specialist Advanced nurse/midwife practitioner (Research)		**Third level** College lecturer Statutory lecturer Senior lecturer Associate professor Professor (Research)	**Centre of nurse education/centre of midwife education (CNE/CME)** Clinical placement coordinator Practice development coordinator Tutor Director of CNE/CME (Research)	Clinical nurse manager 1/clinical midwife manager 1 (CNM1/CMM1) Clinical nurse manager 2/clinical midwife manager 2 (CNM2/CMM2) Clinical nurse manager 3/clinical midwife manager 3 (CNM3/CMM3) Nurse/midwife manager Director of nursing/midwifery
Other roles	**Clinical (hospital and community)**		**Management (hospital and community)**		
Primary care	Registered nurse (general, psychiatric, intellectual disability, children's) Palliative nurse Registered midwife Public health nurse Practice nurse (Research)		Assistant director of public health nursing Director of public health nursing		
Joint appointments	Clinical/academic joint appointments in nursing and midwifery				

Other role development opportunities for nurses and midwives include posts in areas of policy development such as:

- Chief nursing officer in the Department of Health and Children
- Nurse advisors in the Department of Health and Children
- Chief education officer in An Bord Altranais
- Education officers in An Bord Altranais
- Chief executive of the National Council
- Head of professional development and continuing education in the National Council
- Professional development officers in the National Council
- Director of nursing services in the Health Service Executive (HSE)
- Directors of the NMPDUs
- Professional development officers in NMPDUs, responsible for such areas as personnel planning and development of educational services.

There are also many nurses in acute, community care and specialised settings involved in quality development and quality assurance roles. Career pathways provide nurses and midwives with clear choices in relation to the development of their careers within the health services. It is important, however, to distinguish this from the more dynamic requirement for role development that responds to changes in health service needs.

Professor Sir George Castledine[54] notes that nurses have been taking on expanded and extended roles in clinical practice for many years. In Ireland the expansion of practice is governed by the *Scope of Nursing and Midwifery Practice Framework*, published by An Bord Altranais,[55] which came about as a result of a demand for guidance in the context of the increasing diversity of practice due to the introduction of the clinical career pathway and of the demands and expectations that were being put on nurses and midwives in clinical practice. The model of clinical career pathway adopted in Ireland (generalist – specialist – advanced practice) is not dissimilar to the Castledine Specialist Career Model,[56] which is based on the identification of four domains of nursing: general, specialist, higher level or advanced, and paramedical. Seven stages of specialist practice are identified and are each characterised by a description of the achievements expected at each stage.

In progressing along the stages of specialist practice, Castledine pointed to the danger of neglecting the basic nursing principles. The nurse's role, at whatever skill level or mode of specialist functioning, is to help patients with their fundamental nursing needs. As nursing becomes more technical and specialised, there is the danger that it can be taken up with technical outputs and medical targets rather than addressing the basic needs of the patient, which is at the core of nursing.

In Ireland, the National Council has defined the criteria and competencies for recognition at each stage along the career pathway in the form of a framework for the establishment of posts at clinical specialist and advanced practice levels.[57] The National Council has also defined the educational achievements that are required for recognition of post-holders at each level of practice,[58] and provided guidelines for the development of appropriate educational programmes. In addition, the National Council has published a number of position papers on the development of specialist and advanced practitioner roles in emergency departments,[59] intellectual disability services[60] and in older persons nursing.[61] These position papers provide detailed guidance on the assessment of service need and on the approach to be adopted in determining the need. The guidance provided on service needs analysis augments that already provided in the National Council publication *Service Needs Analysis for Clinical Nurse/Midwife Specialists and Advanced Nurse/Midwife Practitioners,*[62] which provides advice and a template for the preparation of a business case to support the development of new roles.

Third-level educational institutions have responded to the development of specialism and advanced practice in nursing and midwifery in Ireland through the development of appropriate courses at postgraduate level. The National Council has worked closely with these institutions in this task. A good example of this can be seen in the collaborative development of a masters' degree course aimed at preparing Ireland's first AMPs.[63] A consultative, collaborative process, involving thirty-eight midwives across Ireland, generated the philosophy, aims and content of the course. The key message was the emphasis on normality rather than specialisation in the development of AMPs.

The development of clinical career pathways has also brought to the fore the increasing importance of research in nursing and midwifery. In 2006, the National Council published a report[64] that provides a picture of nursing and midwifery research activity in Ireland for the period December 2002 to October 2004. A number of proposed actions support the recommendations of the *Research Strategy for Nursing and Midwifery in Ireland*.[65] Other recommendations are set out for building upon the baseline established by this project. A study to identify research priorities for nursing and midwifery in Ireland was carried out in 2005.[66]

The development of nurse-/midwife-led initiatives and the development of the roles of the staff nurse/midwife, the CNS/CMS and the ANP/AMP have the potential to make a major contribution to the implementation of the health service reforms. This is recognised in the key reform documents, in particular in the health strategy *Quality and Fairness: A Health System for You*[67] and the *Report of the National Task Force on Medical Staffing* (known as the *Hanly Report*).[68] The latter comments that the role of the CNS/CMS is already well defined and sits well with the overall recommendation that the skills of health care professionals should be used to best effect. In a response to the *Hanly Report*, the nursing policy division in the Department of Health and Children published *The Challenges for Nursing and Midwifery: A Discussion Paper*.[69] The NMPDU in the former Mid-Western Health Board published a full report[70] on the experiences of two regional pilot sites chosen for reconfiguration of their services in line with the proposals contained in the *Hanly Report*. It included details of the experiences of running nurse-led clinics in the area.

The implementation of the European Working Time Directive (EWTD) in relation to reducing non-consultant hospital doctors' (NCHDs) hours will provide further opportunities for role development. The national implementation group – NIG-EWTD – was set up in early 2005 and is chaired by Dr Cillian Twomey. The multidisciplinary group has approved over twenty pilot projects across all specialties. The NIG-EWTD nursing and midwifery sub-group was set up in early 2005. (The terms 'interdisciplinary' and 'multidisciplinary' are used synonymously throughout this book.)

The National Council has published *An Evaluation of the Effectiveness of the Role of the Clinical Nurse/Midwife Specialist in Ireland*,[71] which demonstrated that there was overwhelming support for the role of the CNS/CMS. The National Council also published *A Preliminary Evaluation of the Role of the Advanced Nurse Practitioner*.[72] Although limited because of the size of the sample involved, this evaluation provided preliminary evidence that ANP roles enhanced patient/client care by providing a holistic service that improved access to health care for patients/clients. They have also been widely accepted by patients/clients, nurses, doctors and other members of the multidisciplinary team.

The changes introduced by the Commission on Nursing in relation to the clinical career pathway have led to a radical transformation of the professions. This transformation, however, will take time to produce the outcomes that are needed. The first degree-qualified cohort of nurses/midwives emerged from the education system in 2006. As yet, it is too early to assess the long-term impact of the changes in the way in which nurses and midwives are being educated.

Building on these changes, the HSE's *Transformation Programme 2007–2010*[73] envisages a crucial role for the staff nurse/midwife, the CNS/CMS and the ANP/AMP. Many other changes are taking place in the role of nurses and midwives throughout the services, including nurse-/midwife-led services and the prescribing of medications.

Nurse-/Midwife-Led Services

As the role of nurses and midwives develops, there has been an increase in the requirement for, and the provision of, a wide range of nurse- and midwife-led services.

Nurse-/midwife-led care is distinct from nurse-/midwife-coordinated or nurse-/midwife-managed services. An evaluation of the extent of nurse-/midwife-led services by the National Council, published in 2005,[74] stated that care is provided by nurses or midwives responsible for case management, the term 'case management' denoting comprehensive patient/client assessment; developing, implementing and managing a plan of care; clinical leadership; and a decision to admit or discharge. Patients/clients will be referred to nurse-/midwife-led services by nurses, midwives or other health care professionals, in accordance with collaboratively agreed protocols.

This care requires enhanced skills and knowledge and the nurse or midwife will need preparation in both the clinical and management aspects of the role. Such nurses or midwives will be practising at an advanced level and may be working in approved specialist or advanced practice roles. Appendix 3 lists the types of nurse-/midwife-led services that have been introduced in Ireland and the number of years they have been established. Appendix 4 lists the types of services that directors of nursing and midwifery intend to introduce in the future.

The issue of nurse-/midwife-led services is one that arises also in relation to the establishment of interdisciplinary teams and the relationships between acute, primary, care and specialised settings but it is not a new concept in health care. In the UK, the National Health Service (NHS) plan for investment and reform,[75] published in 2000, was explicit about the importance of nurse-led services based on the autonomy of the professions. The plan said that the old hierarchical ways of working were giving way to more flexible teamworking involving different clinical professionals. It identified a number of key roles for nurses and midwives:

- Ordering diagnostic investigations, such as pathology tests and X-rays
- Making and receiving referrals
- Admitting and discharging patients with specific conditions within agreed protocols
- Managing caseloads of patients with certain conditions (e.g. diabetes or rheumatology)
- Prescribing medicines and treatments
- Carrying out a wide range of resuscitation procedures including defibrillation
- Performing minor surgery and outpatient procedures
- Triaging patients using the latest information technology
- Taking a lead in the way local health services are organised and managed.

Many of these functions already exist in some services in Ireland and are envisaged as part of the more widespread changes that need to take place within the health services in Ireland in line with the HSE's transformation programme.

A staff nurse or staff midwife who chooses to remain in the clinical area can continue to practise as a staff nurse/midwife and develop his or her role in line with the provisions of the *Scope of Nursing and Midwifery Practice Framework*[76] and the *Guidelines for Midwives*,[77] published by An Bord Altranais. Both the *Scope* and the *Guidelines* documents provide nurses and midwives with a framework to develop their role with considerable scope for flexibility in the interpretation and focus of that role. These guidelines serve to empower nurses and midwives. The scope of nursing and midwifery practice is defined as the range of roles, functions, responsibilities and activities in which a registered nurse/midwife is educated and competent and has authority to perform. The framework was informed by consideration of national and international developments in nursing practice and its aim is to support nurses in the expansion of their scope of practice.

Role development in line with the *Scope* and the *Guidelines* must be supported, however, by a programme of continuing professional development (CPD). A National Council publication, *Report on the Continuing Professional Development of Staff Nurses and Staff Midwives*,[78] published in 2004, linked the demand for role development with the requirement for a lifelong commitment to CPD. Subsequent reports have re-emphasised and strengthened the rationale for improving the way health care is delivered, given the fundamental requirement for accountability and the growing demands to deliver value for money and high-quality service to the consumer. Staff nurses and staff midwives are integral to this process of health service-wide change. Employers, through appropriate education and training needs analysis, can ensure that relevant professional development activities will be provided in a responsive, planned, coherent and equitable manner.

The principal recommendations of the National Council's *Report on the Continuing Professional Development of Staff Nurses and Staff Midwives*[79] were:

- Health service providers should ensure that provision of CPD is based on an education and training needs analysis, a fair and equitable distribution and a policy-based approach to applying for funding.
- Line managers should ensure that job descriptions are competency-based, that part-time and job-sharing staff

become a targeted group for career planning, that orientation programmes are provided and that nurses and midwives are encouraged to engage in professional development planning and the use of portfolios. In addition, peer-focused learning activities should be planned.

- Education providers have a role to play in ensuring fair and equitable provision of CPD opportunities. Access to these programmes should be facilitated through web-based programmes, teleconferencing and modular education programmes. Centres of nurse education (CNEs) and centres of midwife education (CMEs) have a major role in planning and delivery of in-service training and education.
- Individual nurses and midwives have a professional responsibility to engage in CPD activities. This should include the use of personal professional portfolios. They should also be involved in and contribute to ongoing analysis of education and training needs.

In 2005, the National Council conducted a preliminary qualitative evaluation of the role of the ANP.[80] The sample of ANPs used in the evaluation was small, due to the fact that only a limited number of ANPs were actually in post at the time. The evaluation showed that, where they have been introduced, the roles have been successful. The roles are spread over a wide variety of care areas, indicating that roles have developed in response to health service need. The strong clinical focus of the ANP role identified in the study suggests that one of the original aims of the Commission on Nursing, namely, the retention of expert nurses in direct patient care, has been achieved. At the time of writing, the National Council is planning to undertake a more comprehensive and in-depth evaluation of ANP/AMP (and CNS/CMS) roles that should yield more robust evidence about the effectiveness of their clinical interventions and the cost-effectiveness of the services they provide.

The *Agenda for the Future Professional Development of Nursing and Midwifery*,[81] published by the National Council in 2003, highlighted areas for development within the nursing and midwifery professions for general, specialist and advanced practice. To date, many specialist roles in nursing and midwifery have developed around symptom management, diseases, treatments and health promotion. There are opportunities to identify other areas for specialist practice within nursing and midwifery that support holistic practice and enhance continuity of care. For example, areas such as intensive care units (ICUs) have not yet developed CNS roles. The *Agenda* noted that access by nurses and patients to consultation, education and specialist or advanced expertise was limited and the clinical career pathway of nurses and midwives was restricted. A CNS/CMS or ANP/AMP could provide a consultative role, lead and undertake audit, be an educator and carry his or her own caseload. Specialist and advanced practice roles should be considered in all areas of nursing and midwifery practice where there is an identified health service need.

The *Agenda* went on to identify how the role of the nurse and midwife could be developed in each of the branches of the professions, providing specialist nursing/midwifery services in a manner that reflects current health policy and responds to the needs of patients and clients. It stated that any developments should occur within an integrated service development framework and as part of an interdisciplinary approach to service delivery.

The changes in the health system are taking place in accordance with the four guiding principles of the health strategy: better health for everyone; fair access; responsive care delivery; and high performance. In particular, the development of a quality culture throughout the health system can ensure the provision of homogeneous, high-quality, integrated health care at local, regional and national levels. This involves an interdisciplinary approach and continuous evaluation of the system using techniques such as a clinical audit. It also means that information systems must have the capacity to provide feedback to health providers and consumers on the quality of care delivered and received.

The national health strategy, *Quality and Fairness*,[82] stated that professional barriers and structures, job specialisation and the absence of interdisciplinary teams were identified as hindering the integration of services for patients and clients and preventing patients' needs being addressed in an integrated and holistic way. The health strategy was clear in its message: the focus needs to be placed on promoting and facilitating the delivery of health care through interprofessional partnership for the benefit of the patient. The need for an interdisciplinary team approach applied not only to acute services, but also to primary care services. It was not surprising, therefore, that an interdisciplinary national primary care task force was established to drive the implementation of the primary care strategy.

The *Audit of Structures and Functions in the Health System, 2003* report, known as the *Prospectus Report,*[83] also comments on the need for more integration within the health system, commenting that achieving effective integration of services is ultimately a managerial function combined with effective teamworking and interprofessional relationships.

Nurse and Midwife Prescribing

The involvement of nurses and midwives in prescribing is a logical extension of all the other changes in the delivery of services that have been highlighted in this book and of the role that nurses and midwives are expected to play within the services. A national study by the National Council and An Bord Altranais was conducted on the involvement of nurses and midwives in the prescribing of medicines. The final report[84] of the study team recommended that prescriptive authority should be extended to nurses and midwives, subject to regulation. Legislation to enable nurses and midwives to prescribe has now been published. A nurse or midwife who completes the An Bord Altranais-approved prescribing education programme and meets the conditions emanating from the legal regulations may apply to An Bord Altranais to be registered in the new division as a registered nurse prescriber (RNP).[85] The issue of prescription of medication raises the further question of the involvement of nurses and midwives in ordering radiology and laboratory services. Legislation is being finalised at the time of writing to enable nurses, midwives and other professions to order radiology services.

Management in Nursing and Midwifery

The Commission on Nursing highlighted the importance of the role of management in nursing and midwifery. As a result of the recommendations of the Commission, much work has been done in recent years on identifying the key competencies that are required of nurse and midwife managers. The Office for Health

Management (OHM) (whose functions have now been integrated into the HSE's performance and development unit) has been instrumental in the past in health care leadership and management training for professional and non-professional groups within the health service, including nurses and midwives. Specific initiatives included the preparation of personal development plans; a nursing competency framework; a mentoring programme; and the clinicians in management initiative.

In 2000, the OHM published a research report[86] on nursing management competencies. The initiative was based on a recommendation from the Commission on Nursing that competency-based approaches to management should focus on the personal characteristics, skills and behaviours that underpin effective or superior performance. The report set out to identify and define the competencies that were required for effective nursing management in the Irish health and personal social services; to ensure that the competencies were defined in the light of future service requirements and the transitional challenges that they would pose; and to recommend how these management competencies might be applied to enhance the future performance of nursing services. The report identified twenty-one competencies and divided them into four categories: (1) top level competencies, such as strategic, visionary thinking and working at a corporate level, (2) mid-level and (3) front-line competencies, including setting and managing performance standards and building and leading a team, and (4) generic competencies, such as building and maintaining relationships, communication and influencing skills.

A management development sub-group, which played a key role in leadership for managers, was established in 2000 and made further contributions to the enhancement of nursing and midwifery management. The group's initiatives included:

- Providing management development programmes for clinical nurse/midwife managers, CNM2s and CNM3s from 2001 to 2002
- The publication of a guide on commissioning management development programmes for front-line and middle management in 2002
- The delivery and evaluation of the Leading an Empowered Organisation (LEO) programme for CNM1s in three health boards in 2003[87]

- Publishing a diagnostic exercise on the development needs of directors of nursing/equivalent in 2003.[88]

In December 2004, the OHM published a directory of competency development options, which was intended to complement the existing competency-related tools and initiatives for managers in all disciplines within the health services. This included a management competency user pack for nurse and midwife managers,[89] to assist employers and managers in raising understanding of the competencies required at this level and to give practical guidance on how these competencies could be developed and enhanced. One of the flagship programmes of the OHM has been the leadership development programme. This is a multidisciplinary programme that has been running since 1998 and 167 health service employees participated in 2006, including a number of nurse and midwife managers.[90]

Pre-Registration Education

The *Report of the Commission on Nursing* recommended that pre-registration nurse and midwife education should in future be at degree level. The introduction of degree-based pre-registration education for nurses and midwives in Ireland has raised a number of issues that require further discussion. One such issue is the advisability of moving towards a common point of entry for the professions versus the maintenance of the current system based on five different points of entry, and an assessment of the implications of the Bologna Declaration[91] (the joint declaration by the European Ministers of Education, see Appendix 7) for pre-registration nursing and midwifery education in Ireland.

The introduction of a common point-of-entry system for nursing and midwifery in Ireland would be in line with existing systems in the UK and most other countries with a degree programme for pre-registration nurse education. The common point of entry would entail all nurse and midwife students sharing a common first year or eighteen months at university and then choosing to specialise in a particular branch. The advantages of such a system would be the creation of greater intradisciplinary solidarity within the professions and the development of common standards across all the branches of the professions. As it stands, Ireland is the only country that has five separate degree programmes (general, children's, psychiatric and intellectual disability nursing and midwifery). This is not likely to be sustainable in the future.

In June 2004, An Bord Altranais commissioned what became known as the *Five Points Project*[92] to examine the rationale for and impact of maintaining the five points of entry. The study concluded with a series of recommendations that summarise the overall approach to pre-registration entry to nursing and midwifery education prevailing in Ireland today. The Bologna Declaration will take effect in 2010 and will involve a change to a three-year degree programme, followed by a year of internship. This will have significant implications for clinical placements and other elements of the current four-year degree programme.

Is this an opportune time to conduct an evaluation of the whole programme? Such a review would present the opportunity to re-examine options such as a single point of entry to nursing and midwifery, shared common basic education for nursing and midwifery students, and the advisability or otherwise of sharing some education with other third-level students in areas such as science, medicine and other health disciplines.

In July 2007, it was reported[93] that the Department of Health and Children was to commission a review of the current nursing and midwifery degree programmes with a view to determining whether the investment in these programmes has represented value for money for the taxpayer. In making the announcement, the Minister for Health and Children, Mary Harney, TD, said that to date over €700 million had been spent on the degree programme since 2002.

Some concern has been voiced about the advisability of conducting a full-scale value for money review just one year after the first cohort of degree students has graduated.[94] A value for money analysis of its very nature considers quantitative data such as inputs and outputs as a measure of economy and efficiency. An example of a quantitative study[95] on the effects of levels of nursing education on patient outcomes can be found in the United States, which set out to determine whether the educational levels of registered nurses in hospitals had a measurable effect on patient outcomes. It found that a 10 per cent increase in the proportion of nurses holding a bachelor's degree was associated with a 5 per cent decrease in both the likelihood of patients dying within thirty days of admission and the odds of failure to rescue. The conclusion of the study was that in hospitals with higher proportions of nurses educated at the baccalaureate level or higher, surgical patients experienced lower mortality and failure to rescue rates.

It is too early as yet to determine whether the degree programme in Ireland has had any impact on the delivery of services in Ireland. It could also be argued that a full analysis of the impact of the degree programme would require a review based on qualitative data such as patient satisfaction, quality of care and other non-quantitative criteria. Any review of pre-registration nursing and midwifery education, however, would necessarily have to look in detail at the benefits and opportunities presented by common point of entry and interdisciplinary education.

Post-Registration Education

In January 2007, the HSE established a post-registration nursing and midwifery education review group (PRERG) to prepare a comprehensive strategy for the development, delivery and evaluation of future post-registration nursing and midwifery education. The group will examine the need for the provision of post-registration programmes leading to registration with An Bord Altranais and is expected to publish an overarching framework for the development of future post-registration programmes, including a preferred model for procuring and financing the development and delivery of these programmes. The PRERG put forward a series of recommendations in the areas of practice, education, policy and research based on the literature review undertaken by the Catherine McAuley School of Nursing, University College Cork, on behalf of the group.[96]

Continuing Professional Development

The National Council defines continuing professional development (CPD) as:

> ...a lifelong process, which includes both structured and informal activities that may include formal education programmes, participation in journal clubs, case conferencing, clinical supervision, learning sets, preceptorship, mentorship, workshops, distance learning

> programmes and reflection on practice. CPD encompasses processes, activities and experiences that contribute towards the development of a nurse or midwife, both personally and professionally.[97]

Further, the National Council has adopted the definition of the related concept of lifelong learning as a continuously supportive process which stimulates and empowers individuals to acquire all the knowledge, values, skills and understanding they will require throughout their lifetimes, and to apply them with competence, creativity and enjoyment in all roles, circumstances and environments.[98]

The National Council refers to what are called the components and attributes of competence resulting in effective and/or superior performance. These include practical and technical skills, communication and interpersonal skills, organisational and managerial skills, the ability to practice safely and effectively, utilising evidence-based practice, having a problem-solving approach to care, utilising critical thinking, being part of a multidisciplinary team, demonstrating a professional attitude, accepting responsibility, and being accountable for one's practice.

One of the factors impeding participation in CPD by all nurses and midwives is access. Nurses and midwives living and working in more remote areas of the country may find it difficult to get time off to attend educational courses and activities that are held in centres that are far from their place of work. One possible solution is electronic learning or e-learning: web-based initiatives designed to provide access to CPD opportunities. The 'eLearning Guru'[99] provided by the HSE performance and development website describes a wide range of advantages inherent in this approach.

The National Council has adopted some of the principles of e-learning as part of its overall communications strategy, by providing access to a wide range of learning opportunities on its website (e.g. the medication management programme) and by hosting websites of specialist groups and learning initiatives within nursing and midwifery. The website also contains links to databases such as the all-Ireland practice and quality development database, developed in partnership between the National Council and the Northern Ireland Practice and Education Council (NIPEC).

The importance of CPD in the lives of nurses and midwives was one of the motivating factors behind the publication by the National Council of *Guidelines for Portfolio Development for Nurses and Midwives.*[100] The guidelines are aimed at individual nurses and midwives working at the forefront of health care delivery, to assist them to identify, reflect upon and record the contribution they make to direct and indirect care, encourage them to store records of their development in a coherent and structured manner and provide guidance and information on achieving their individual professional goals within the context of the needs of the health service.

The National Council has an important role to play in providing nurses and midwives with additional continuing education opportunities that enhance their ability to maximise their potential in their chosen clinical career pathway. Between 2001 and 2007 the National Council disbursed a total of €16 million to fund 769 initiatives, such as professional and service developments, courses, seminars and workshops. Over 27,000 nurses and midwives have benefited directly and indirectly from these initiatives.

The National Council has published three reports on the future professional development of nursing and midwifery:

- *Agenda for the Future Professional Development of Nursing and Midwifery.*[101] The National Council conducted a nationwide consultation from March 2002 to March 2003. Workshops were held with directors of nursing and midwifery, directors of the NMPDUs, and nurses and midwives from all divisions of the Register. A call for submissions yielded 105 written responses. The report benchmarks progress to date for general, mental health, children's, intellectual disability and older person nursing and midwifery and sets the agenda for a debate on options, direction and actions for the future. CPD emerges as the predominant issue in this report for all areas of nursing and is viewed as vital to developing nursing and midwifery practice in modern health structures.
- *Report on the Continuing Professional Development of Staff Nurses and Staff Midwives.*[102] This report reviewed CPD activities of staff nurses and midwives; competency achievements and maintenance relevant to service need and

personal professional development; and the career choices relevant to CPD and competency of staff nurses and staff midwives. The data collection methods for this report included a literature review, focus groups and a questionnaire. Staff nurses from general, mental health, intellectual disability and children's nursing and staff midwives were invited to participate. Nurses and midwives from cities, towns and rural areas were represented, as were those working in community and in-patient settings. Recommendations covered the development of structures to support CPD for staff nurses and staff midwives. The report contained a detailed table of recommendations that summarised the objectives, the deliverables and the responsibilities of individual stakeholders in this area.

- *Agenda for the Future Professional Development of Public Health Nursing.*[103] A nationwide consultation was carried out from November 2004 to February 2005. Workshops were held with directors of public health nursing, assistant directors of public health nursing, public health nurses engaged in clinical practice and other key stakeholders. The main concerns expressed by participants related to role clarity, workload demands, variation in service provision and delivery of care, the clinical career pathway, leadership, skill mix and multidisciplinary team working. The report benchmarked progress on professional development to date and set an agenda for future actions.

Joint Appointments

The Commission on Nursing mentioned the potential offered by the use of joint appointments between clinical and academic institutions. A separate publication was prepared on the subject in line with the recommendations of the Commission.[104] In 2005, the National Council published a report[105] on joint appointments that provides a framework for institutions and individuals involved in making joint appointments between services, voluntary organisations, educational institutions and/or other organisations. Joint appointments require careful planning and support mechanisms.

The Office for Public Management has produced a *Joint Appointments Guide*,[106] which provides guidance on setting up, managing and maintaining joint appointments for health improvement between health organisations and local government. The guide identified the importance of strategic planning as a key to success, indicating that the critical success factors were early planning and clear strategic purpose. There is potential for the creation of a nursing equivalent of the 'clinician scientist'. This is something that is used in medicine, whereby an individual works within the clinical area with a clinical caseload, but whose main focus is the development of research. Appointments such as these are promoted and funded by the Health Research Board. There would appear to be opportunities for similar positions to be created in nursing and midwifery.

Conclusions

The following conclusions can be drawn from the discussion presented in this chapter:

- The five points of entry to nursing and midwifery in Ireland will need to be reviewed in the light of the requirements of the Bologna Declaration and of international best practice. The demands of the service for an integrated approach to service delivery would also suggest that a single point of entry based on interdisciplinary approaches to education and training of nurses and midwives would be desirable.
- In developing the clinical career pathway for nurses and midwives particular attention needs to be given to maintaining the integrity of the professions. This entails recognising the prime importance of the generalist nurse and midwife engaging in direct provision of care to individuals in need. Development of specialties and advanced practice should support this key role and add value to the core functions of nursing and midwifery.
- The nursing and midwifery professions have an important role to play in achieving efficiency and effectiveness gains in the reform of the health services. It is important that, in achieving this, the professions develop in line with their core values and identity.

- The use of joint appointments between clinical and educational settings should be extended in order to emphasise the importance of the frontline clinical role of the nurse and midwife in providing care.
- Nurses and midwives should be encouraged to develop and lead services in both acute and primary care settings in a way that is responsive to the needs of patients and clients. Nursing and midwifery management should provide the necessary leadership to make this possible, by empowering and encouraging individual nurses in this way.
- Nurses and midwives should be facilitated and encouraged to engage in continuing professional development, promoting a culture of a lifelong commitment to learning. Consideration should be given to ways of demonstrating this commitment by providing evidence as a condition of continuing registration.

CHAPTER 3

A Changing Society and its Implications for Nursing and Midwifery

Nursing and midwifery in Ireland operate within a health care environment that is influenced by social, economic, demographic and epidemiological factors. This environment is also influenced by policy responses to the needs of the population and the growing demands of the health services. A brief review follows of key factors that are likely to impact on the development of a strategy for the future of the professions.

Population and Economic Change

The impact of the so-called Celtic Tiger economic boom of the past decade is frequently reported as having transformed Ireland, with both positive and negative social consequences. A recent book, *Best of Times? The Social Impact of the Celtic Tiger,*[107] which brought together the work of social researchers from the Economic and Social Research Institute (ESRI), National University of Ireland, Maynooth (NUI Maynooth), and University College Dublin (UCD), concluded that the social impact of progress has been largely positive, resulting in a decline in poverty rates, increased social mobility and improvements in the health of the nation.

The downturn in the Irish economy, experienced in 2008, is expected to be short-term. The ESRI forecasts[108] that the economy is set to recover rapidly, with continuing medium-term growth above the EU average. The Central Statistics Office's (CSO) third report in the series *Measuring Ireland's Progress*[109] provided a detailed analysis of Ireland's situation in respect of key economic, social and statistical indicators in comparison with other European Union (EU) countries. The report confirms that Ireland has experienced extraordinary growth in population and in the economy in recent years. The following facts and statistics paint a picture of a country that has experienced, and is likely to continue to experience, significant change.

- **Population**: The population in Ireland increased by 15.7 per cent to almost 4.24 million persons in the period 1997–2006. The fertility rate in Ireland was the second highest in the EU in 2005, at a rate of 1.88 per woman compared to an EU 25 average of 1.52. Life expectancy at birth was 81.8 years for Irish women and 77.1 years for Irish men in 2005. Life expectancy for men in Ireland was 1.3 years above the EU 25 average of 75.8 years, while that for women was 0.1 years below the EU 25 average of 81.9 years.
- **GDP**: In 2005, Ireland had the second highest Gross Domestic Product (GDP) per capita within the EU 25, expressed in terms of purchasing power standards, at 38.9 per cent above the EU average. Based on Gross National Income (GNI), Ireland was in fifth place at 18.6 per cent above the EU average. Investment in Ireland in Gross Fixed Capital Formation (GFCF) increased by almost 43 per cent over the period 1996–2005. In each year since 1997 Ireland has invested a higher proportion of GDP in GFCF than the EU average.
- **Health care spending**: An average of €2,223 (at constant 2003 prices) per person was spent on non-capital public expenditure on health care in Ireland in 2004. This was an increase of over 80 per cent on the 1995 level.
- **Education spending**: Non-capital public expenditure on education per student rose by 45.2 per cent between 1996 and 2005, after allowing for inflation. Most of the increased expenditure was directed towards primary and secondary education.
- **Schooling**: The pupil–teacher ratio at primary level in Ireland in the school year 2003–2004 was one of the highest in the EU 27 at 18:3; 12 of the other 26 EU member states had a pupil–teacher ratio of less than 15:1 at primary level. Early school leavers represented 12.3 per cent of the 18–24 age group in Ireland in 2006. The unemployment rate for early school leavers in this age group was 19 per cent in 2006 compared with an unemployment rate of 8.2 per cent for all persons aged 18–24.
- **Ageing**: According to CSO projections,[110] the older population (i.e. those aged 65 years and over) will increase from its 2001 level of 430,000 to over 1.1 million by 2036. The

very old population (i.e. those aged 80 years and over) is set to rise even more dramatically, from the 2001 level of 98,000 to a projected 323,000 in 2036. The average annual number of deaths will increase steadily, from a current figure of fewer than 30,000, to over 40,000 in the period 2031–2036. The natural increase in the population (i.e. the excess of births over deaths) is projected to decline; however, it will remain positive over the course of the projection period (2006–2036). The young population (827,500) was almost double the old population (430,000) in 2001. However, by 2036 it is projected that there will be more older persons than younger persons (i.e. 1,119,000 persons aged 65 years and over compared with just 750,000 persons aged 0–14 years).

- **Immigration**: There was a 53 per cent increase in the immigrant population between 2002 and 2006 and foreign-born residents accounted for 14 per cent of the population in 2006, compared with 10 per cent in 2002. Non-Irish nationals accounted for one in eight workers in the state and one in three workers in the hotel and restaurant sector in 2006. More than a quarter of the population of large areas of Dublin are immigrants.[111]
- **Employment**: The employment rate in Ireland rose from 56.1 per cent in 1997 to 68.1 per cent in 2006. The rate for women in employment increased by over 14 per cent over that period, while the rate for men rose by around 10 per cent. Productivity in Ireland, measured as GDP per person employed, was the second highest in the EU 27 in 2005. The unemployment rate in Ireland increased from a low point of 3.6 per cent in 2001 to 4.3 per cent in 2006. Ireland had the third lowest unemployment rate in the EU 27 in 2006 at just over half of the EU average of 7.9 per cent. The long-term unemployment rate in Ireland was 1.4 per cent in 2005, which was lower than the EU 27 average of 4 per cent. The employment rate of persons aged 55–64 at 51.7 per cent was higher than the EU 27 average of 42.3 per cent in 2005. However, only 37.4 per cent of women in Ireland in this age group were in employment compared to 65.7 per cent of men.
- **Labour force**: There has been a 17 per cent increase in the number of people in the labour force in the past four years. Agriculture accounted for less than 5 per cent of total

employment in 2006, compared with over 50 per cent in 1926. Female labour force participation increased sharply from 29.7 per cent in 1981 to 52.8 per cent in 2006. The percentage of women describing themselves as homemakers, staying at home, fell from 54.9 per cent in 1981 to 21.8 per cent in 2006.[112]
- **Carers**: There were almost 161,000 unpaid carers in the State in 2006, just under 5 per cent of the population. Women accounted for 62 per cent of carers with most of them aged in their forties or fifties.[113]
- **Poverty**: Over 6 per cent of men and 7.5 per cent of women in Ireland were in consistent poverty in 2005, with unemployed people most likely to be in consistent poverty. The proportion of Irish people at risk of poverty, after pensions and social transfer payments were taken into account, was 20 per cent in 2005. This was one of the highest rates in the EU 27. The effect of pensions and social transfers on reducing the at-risk-of-poverty rate was low in Ireland compared with other EU 27 countries. In 2004, social protection expenditure in Ireland was 17 per cent of GDP.

It is apparent from these statistics that Ireland has become a wealthy country in a relatively short period of time and the Government has stated that it is investing in social services, such as education and health, at an increased rate compared to the past. This would indicate a country that is in transition as it seeks to build up its capital infrastructure in key social services. Problems arising from social exclusion and poverty continue to be significant. The growth in population and, in particular, the major increase in the multi-cultural and multi-ethnic make-up of the population and of the workforce present challenges for all service planners and service deliverers, and those in the health services. These challenges include the ability to adapt to more diverse cultural contexts and avoid specifically multi-cultural barriers within health service delivery.

While Ireland has a relatively young population at present compared to other EU countries, the prospects are for a notable increase in the number of older people. The ageing of the population over the next twenty to thirty years will change the level of dependency that exists within the country and will require the creation of services to cater for the needs of an increased number of older people.

There continues to be greater participation by women in the labour force and this has implications for the shaping of the primary health care provisions of the future, the aspirations of which are frequently based on a traditional view of what the family framework is likely to be. There is a need to look again at the support that is given to families and carers in their own homes, and take account of the changing nature of 'family frameworks'.

The Health Services

Like the economy and the rest of Irish society, Irish health services are currently in transition. Some of the key features of relevance to the health services are summarised in the following facts and statistics:[114]

- **Employment**: The number of people employed in the health services in Ireland in December 2006 was 106,273. Table 2 provides a summary of the different grades of staff employed in the health services at that time.

Table 2: Employment in Health Services in Ireland, 2006[115]

Nurses	36,737	35%
Medical/Dental	7,712	7%
Health and social care professionals	14,913	14%
Other patient and client care staff	16,739	16%
Management and administration	17,262	16%
General support staff	12,910	12%
Total	106,273	100%

- **Doctors and nurses**: In June 2008, the Organisation for Economic Co-operation and Development (OECD) published statistics on health care in member countries that contained key facts on resource levels within the health services in Ireland.[116] Despite increasing numbers of doctors in recent years, Ireland continues to have fewer physicians per capita than many other OECD countries. In 2006, Ireland had 2.9 physicians per 1,000 head of population, compared with an OECD average of 3.1. While the number of doctors per capita in Ireland is higher than in the UK, the United States, Canada and Australia, it is lower than in a number of other European countries. On the other hand, Ireland has a very high proportion of practising nurses, with 15.4 nurses per 1,000 head of population in 2006, compared with an OECD average of 9.7. It is important to note, however, that the comparability of data on nurses is more limited, due to the inclusion of different classes of nurses and midwives in the data reported by different countries.

- **Acute public hospitals**: The ESRI reports[117] that there was a major increase in activity in Irish acute public hospitals for the period 1990–1999. The number of people treated in 1999 increased by over 40 per cent on the figures for 1990 to 800,000. Much of this increase was attributed to reductions in the length of patient/client stays and the increase in the number of day beds in hospitals, which resulted in increased use of day services.
- **Extended care facilities**: The number of beds in extended care facilities in Ireland in 2003 was 23,825. The bed occupancy rate was 88.9 per cent, with a total of 21,169 patients. Of these, 11,486 beds were in private nursing homes, with a bed occupancy rate of 86.8 per cent and a total of 9,965 patients.[118] The number of acute care hospital beds in Ireland in 2005 was 2.8 per 1,000 of population, which was below the OECD average of 3.9 beds per 1,000 of population. In most OECD countries, including Ireland, the number of hospital beds per capita has fallen over time.
- **Mental health**: The number of in-patients in all psychiatric hospitals and units in Ireland at 31 December 2001 and 31 December 2002 were 4,256 and 3,891 respectively. The main focus of care in the mental health services is now in the community as the number of in-patients/clients in psychiatric hospitals has been decreasing over recent years, with the focus of in-patient care being only for short-term acute episodes or for chronically disturbed patients/clients who cannot function in lower support environments. According to statistics published by the Department of Health and Children in 2001, it was estimated at that time that one person in four would suffer from mental illness at some stage during their life, and that one in four families were likely to have at least one member suffering from a mental illness. In addition, the incidence of depression in Ireland was estimated to be 10 per cent of the population and

schizophrenia was 1 per cent.[119] Suicide is strongly related to depression. The number of deaths from suicide has decreased from a high of 478 in 2002 to 409 in 2006.[120]

- **Intellectual disability (ID)**: In April 2007, there were 25,613 people registered on the national intellectual disability database (NIDD) of the Health Research Board (HRB), with a prevalence of 6.04 per 1,000 head of the total population. The prevalence rate for mild ID was 1.96 per 1,000 and the prevalence rate for moderate, severe and profound ID was 3.48 per 1,000 (10 per cent of cases registered on the NIDD in 2007 did not have their degree of intellectual disability confirmed, this represents a prevalence rate of 0.60 per 1,000 head of total population). There were 8,135 people with intellectual disabilities in residential placements in Ireland in 2006. This number increased to 8,210 in 2007. The number of persons availing of day programmes for people with intellectual disabilities in 2006 was 24,386. Of these, 8,044 were in residential placements and 16,342 were day attendees. The corresponding figures for 2007 were 24,729, 8,125 and 16,604.[121]
- **Mortality**: Most people in Ireland today can expect to live into old age. This is in striking contrast to the situation at the beginning of the twentieth century, where life expectancy was around fifty years. According to CSO data,[122] at the end of 2006 the greatest causes of mortality in Ireland were circulatory disease (35 per cent), malignant neoplasms (29 per cent), respiratory diseases (14 per cent), and injuries and poisonings (5 per cent). The overall death rate per 100,000 of population in Ireland has decreased from 1,136.8 in 1972 to 749.2 in 2002. Deaths from circulatory diseases over the same period have declined from 579.6 in 1972 to 296.0 in 2002. Deaths from cancer for the same period have increased from 190.5 in 1972 to 191.4 in 2002. However, in the case of cancer, the death rate in 1992 had increased to 212.1 and has decreased over the following ten years. Deaths from external causes of injury and poisoning have declined over the same period from 55.5 in 1972 to 39.3 in 2002.[123]
- **Lifestyle**: The *National Health and Lifestyle Surveys* monitor lifestyle and health-related indicators. In 1999, the survey reported[124] that 32 per cent of adults were overweight and that exercise was likely to decrease with age. It also reported

that most adults consumed alcohol and that one in four exceeded the recommended weekly limits for sensible drinking. Less healthy lifestyles were observed in lower socioeconomic groups. The second *National Health and Lifestyle Surveys*, published in 2003,[125] found that there had been a 2 per cent drop since 1998 in the percentage of school-age children smoking, particularly in the 12–14 year age group. On alcohol consumption, the survey found that there had been an increase of 9 per cent in the numbers of school-age children who had never consumed an alcoholic drink, this being most marked in 10–11 year olds. The survey reported that rates of obesity had increased by 3 per cent, but the percentage engaging in physical exercise had improved in some age groups. It also reported a strong inverse trend according to educational status at all ages, and only modest drops in rates of smoking. In 2005, the *Report of the National Task Force on Obesity*[126] reported that obesity is now a major public health problem throughout Europe. In Ireland, 39 per cent of adults are overweight and 18 per cent are obese. Of these, slightly more men than women are obese. There is a higher incidence of the disease in the lower socioeconomic groups. The report suggests that the problem is particularly acute in relation to childhood obesity and authoritative estimates put the number of overweight and obese children on the island of Ireland at more than 300,000, with this number rising at a rate of over 10,000 per year.

These statistics show that there has been a major increase in activity within the Irish health services. This is a direct result of the decrease in the length of stay in acute hospitals. This shows a need for a shift to more community-based follow-up care, especially in psychiatric services, where the number of in-patient cases has declined over recent years. An increase in life expectancy means that there will be an increasingly older population and confirms the projections of population growth. The health services will also have to contend with an increase in lifestyle-related illnesses and conditions. As nurses make up the largest group of health care professionals (35 per cent), it is likely that the bulk of health care delivery will fall on this group of professionals.

Conclusions

The following are key conclusions from this element of the review of the changes in Irish society and of the services provided for and needed by particular population groups:

- The health services of the future will be delivered to a population that is generally wealthier, with higher expectations about what they can expect from public services. This will increase pressure for continued investment in both capital and current spending on health services.
- Ireland's population will continue to grow at a fast rate and the birth rate will continue to increase. The number of older people will increase, with implications for dependency relationships from both a social and an economic perspective.
- Increased labour force participation by women, together with an increase in the number of dependent older people, will have implications for the traditional care structures that existed within families. This, in turn, will have implications for the provision of community-based primary care services. The bulk of the demands in this area will fall on nurses and midwives, who make up the largest portion of the labour force in the health services.
- Increased wealth has brought about and will continue to bring with it an increase in lifestyle diseases. Conversely, there will continue to be poverty-related diseases and social problems due to social exclusion and lack of participation.
- The population of Ireland will continue to become more ethnically and culturally diverse. This has significant implications for the delivery of services and, in particular, the need for sensitivity to cultural differences and communications issues. It also raises questions for the recruitment practices within the services and the need for increased training for professionals and administrators in dealing with a more diverse population and consumer base.

CHAPTER 4

Health Service Reform Programme

The Health Service Reform Programme (HSRP) is shaping the future of the Irish health services.[127] The programme is based on the recommendations that emerged from a number of reports that are commonly referred to as the *Prospectus Report*,[128] the *Brennan Report*[129] and the *Hanly Report*.[130] The reports were commissioned following the publication in 2001 of the health strategy *Quality and Fairness: A Health System For You*,[131] and were published in 2003. The key recommendations to emerge concerned:

- A new national management structure for the health service
- A reduction in the number of agencies involved in the planning and delivery of health and personal social services
- New financial accountability systems
- A reconfiguration of hospital services.

In order to understand the implications of the reform programme for the future of the Irish health services, it is important to review the reports on which these recommendations were based.

Health Strategy

All government departments and agencies in Ireland are required to produce three- or five-year strategy documents.[132] The Department of Health and Children's strategy, *Quality and Fairness*, outlined a programme of investment and reform of the health system, which was to be implemented over a ten-year period. It set out four overall national goals:

- Better health for everyone
- Fair access to publicly funded services
- Responsive and appropriate care delivery by an effective and efficient health system
- High performance in terms of quality of care, planning and decision-making, and accountability.

The relevance of the health strategy to nurses and midwives cannot be overstated. Specific nursing roles are mentioned, such as the ANP (Emergency), as are opportunities and supports for professional development.

In keeping with the principle of people-centredness, the strategy refers to the need for integrated, continuous, high-quality services and greater interdisciplinary working. An example of this is the requirement for greater coordination between child welfare and protection, and primary care services such as general practice and public health nursing, and child and adolescent psychiatric teams. This could be a catalyst for nurses working in primary care settings to develop their knowledge of, and skills in, working with children with mental health problems by liaising more closely with nurses working in psychiatric or intellectual disability services.

The health strategy describes the health service workforce as highly committed and dedicated and as having enabled very significant developments to be undertaken. It suggests that this same workforce can overcome obstacles to a more integrated or seamless service through the development and implementation of information technology systems, data and information sharing, and the reduction of the professional and structural barriers. Advances in information and communication technology (ICT) are viewed as likely to revolutionise care. These advances include patient-care databases and opportunities to work to standardised, evidence-based protocols and decision-support systems.

A national goal of the health strategy is responsive and appropriate care delivery and seeks to gear the health system to respond appropriately and adequately to the needs of individuals and families. It is also concerned with ensuring that the various parts of the system are being utilised to their maximum effectiveness and efficiency. Objectives related to this goal include ensuring that the system has the capacity to deliver timely and appropriate services and that the patient is at the centre in the delivery of care. In order to achieve this, the strategy states that an integrated approach to care planning for individuals will become a consistent feature of the system.

A further goal is high performance, which relates to quality of care, planning and decision-making, the efficiency and effectiveness of the system, commitment to continuous improvement and full accountability. The principles of quality and accountability are embraced by the objectives identified under this goal. These objectives are concerned with standardised quality systems to support best patient care and safety, and evidence and strategic objectives to underpin all planning/decision-making. An evidence- based approach to decision-making requires research findings, qualitative and quantitative data, and other documented trends and behaviours.

The Health Service Reform Programme represented the biggest move to reform the health services in Ireland in over thirty years. The last major reform of the health services took place on foot of the *Health Act, 1970,* which saw the introduction of the eight health boards.[133] Over the years since then, a number of initiatives took place, the most important of which have been:[134]

- 1986 ***Health: The Wider Dimensions***.[135] This was in response to the WHO objectives set out in *Health for All by the Year 2000*[136] and represented an attempt to set a new direction for the services in order to achieve these objectives.
- 1989 The ***Commission on Health Funding***[137] provided an analysis of the key faults in the organisation of the health services and examined the financing of the services with recommendations on the future funding required.
- 1990 The ***Dublin hospital initiative group (Kennedy Reports)***.[138] The group was set up to improve the coordination of hospital services and the integration of hospital and other services in the Dublin area. It recommended the setting up of a new authority to replace the Eastern Health Board. It also recommended that the Department of Health should be less involved in the direct management of services and should take a greater role in policy and strategic issues.
- 1994 The ***Health Strategy: Shaping a Healthier Future***[139] was a precursor to the Health Service Reform Programme and focused on the re-orientation and reshaping of the health services so that improving people's health and quality of life became the primary and unifying focus of the health services.
- 1997 The ***Statement of Strategy***[140] was the response by the Department of Health to the strategic management initiative in the civil service.

- 1998 ***Working for Health and Well-Being***.[141] This strategy statement addressed the challenges faced by the Department in service delivery as a result of the *Public Services Management Act, 1997*[142] and the *Freedom of Information Act, 1997*.[143]

Prospectus Report

The primary objective of the *Audit of Structures and Functions in the Health Service*, known as the *Prospectus Report*,[144] was to establish the organisational improvements needed to strengthen the capacity of the health system to meet the challenges of implementing the programme of development and reform set out in the health strategy. The following key reforms were proposed:

- Major rationalisation of existing health service agencies to reduce fragmentation
- Re-organisation of the Department of Health and Children, to ensure improved policy development and oversight
- Establishment of the Health Service Executive (HSE), which would be the first ever body charged with managing the health service as a single national entity
- Establishment of three core areas within the HSE: a National Hospitals' Office (NHO), a primary, community and continuing care directorate (PCCC) and a National Shared Services Centre (NSSC)
- Establishment of four regional health offices within the HSE to deliver regional and local services
- Immediate establishment of an interim National Hospitals' Office (NHO) with the priority of reforming the hospital sector
- Establishment of a Health Information and Quality Authority (HIQA) to ensure that quality of care was promoted throughout the system
- Devolving responsibility for care budgets to the people actually in charge of delivering that care
- Complete modernisation of supporting processes (service planning, management reporting, etc.) to improve planning and delivery of services, including maximising the impact of public funding.

In order to consolidate the system further and reduce the fragmentation that undermines the national management of the system, the report recommended that up to twenty-five existing agencies should be subsumed into the HSE, HIQA or the restructured Department of Health and Children. Another seven bodies should be otherwise merged or abolished.

Brennan Report

The *Report of the Commission on Financial Management and Control Systems in the Health Service*, known as the *Brennan Report*, contains a detailed examination and review of the financial management and control systems in the Irish health service. The Commission found problems in the existing system and adopted four core principles in addressing these problems:

- The health service should be managed as a national system
- Accountability should rest with those who have the authority to commit the expenditure
- All costs incurred should be capable of being allocated to individual patients
- Good financial management and control should not be seen solely as a finance function.

Its recommendations included:

- The establishment of an Executive to manage the Irish health service as a unitary national service
- A range of reforms to governance and financial management, control and reporting systems to support the Executive in the management of the system
- Substantial rationalisation of existing health agencies
- Strengthening the process of evaluation of clinical and cost effectiveness for publicly funded drug schemes
- Pending the establishment of the Executive, the creation of a high-level and well-resourced implementation committee.

There is evidence that the recommendations of the *Brennan Report* are being incorporated into policy and service development. Perhaps the most obvious evidence is the creation of the HSE, involving a complete separation of policy and executive functions and charging the Department of Health and Children with the role of monitoring and evaluating the work of the HSE and its expenditure.

Other practical examples also point to changes in culture. In September 2006, the Department of Health and Children announced the establishment of an inter-agency group, which will seek to ensure value for money on health service projects. The group focused initially on areas such as pharmaceuticals, procurement, estate management, employment management and administrative spending. It also has a role in monitoring adherence to value for money requirements in capital investment expenditure on information and computer technology and on consultancies. Chaired by the secretary general of the Department, membership of the group includes the chief executive officer (CEO) of the HSE, the chief executive of HIQA and a senior official of the Department of Finance. The group is charged with providing a further level of assurance to the Minister for Health and Children, the Department of Finance and the HSE board that value for money in health spending is getting the required attention.

The setting up of this group was directly related to the implementation of the recommendations in the *Brennan Report*. In March 2007, it was reported[145] that the group was seeking savings of €500 million between 2007 and 2010 and that the money thus saved would be ring-fenced for frontline services. The savings were to be made from within the annual budget of the HSE, which amounts to €14 billion per annum.

Hanly Report

The *Report of the National Task Force on Medical Staffing*, known as the *Hanly Report*, was published in 2003. Its purpose was to devise a plan for reducing substantially the average working hours of non-consultant hospital doctors to meet the requirements of the European Working Time Directive (EWTD); to plan for the implementation of a consultant-provided service; and to address the medical education and training needs associated with the EWTD and the move to a consultant-provided service. The report recommended that multidisciplinary working between health and social care professionals should be fostered, and that this would best be achieved through close liaison between the universities at undergraduate level and the relevant professional bodies at postgraduate level. It also proposed introducing or further developing grades of staff that would facilitate a more appropriate distribution of skills and functions. The focus was on grades that would bring genuine opportunities to deliver health care more efficiently, taking account of who should best provide the services required.

In response to the *Hanly Report*, the nursing policy division of the Department of Health and Children produced a discussion paper[146] that outlined the critical success factors necessary for nursing and midwifery to meet the challenges the report presented. These factors included the development of skills over time, partnership, change management and the development of clinical competence guidelines.

HSE

In December 2004, the Minister for Health and Children, Mary Harney, TD, signed the relevant Orders bringing the HSE into operation with effect from 1 January 2005. The basis of the Health Service Reform Programme is the separation of policy formulation from service delivery. The Department would henceforth concentrate on policy formulation and evaluation and the Minister would hold the HSE to account for the delivery, within budget, of publicly funded health services. The HSE would, in turn, manage the health service as a single national entity and would also provide advice to the Minister and contribute to policy formulation.

The organisational structure of the HSE has developed since it was first introduced. As of March 2008, it comprises four divisions: health and personal social services; support structures; the office of the CEO; and reform and innovation. The principle service delivery arm of the HSE is the health and personal social services division, which is divided into what have become known as the three pillars of service delivery:

1. **Population health**, which includes functional units for health protection, health promotion, environmental health, emergency planning, strategic planning and evaluation, health intelligence, and transition and change.
2. **Primary, community and continuing care (PCCC)**, which includes functional units that cover four geographic areas (Dublin Mid-Lenister, Dublin North-East, South and West), each of which, in addition to the management of services

within its own geographic area, has national responsibility for a different area of care (i.e. (1) primary care; (2) children, youth, family, palliative care and chronic illness; (3) older persons and social inclusion; and (4) mental health and disabilities). In addition, PCCC is responsible for thirty-two local health offices, each of which is manned by a local health manager. These local offices are key elements in the management and development of services at a local level. They provide an essential bridge between the national and regional dimensions.

3. **The National Hospitals' Office (NHO)**, which is responsible for the management of the fifty-three hospitals that exist throughout the country. This is done through a group of eight network managers, two in each of the four geographic areas. Each network manager has responsibility for a group of hospital services in his/her area, and, together with the local health managers in PCCC, are key health service development and management stakeholders. In addition, the NHO is responsible for pre-hospital emergency care, which includes the ambulance service; contracts and utilisation; quality, risk and consumer affairs; and planning and development.

The establishment of the HSE has implications for the role of the Department of Health and Children. The role of the Department now is to support the Minister and the democratic process by:

- Formulating policy underpinned by an evidence-based approach and providing direction on national health priorities, ensuring that quality and value for money are enhanced through monitoring and evaluation.
- Protecting the interests of patients and consumers and supporting practitioners and professionals to practise to the highest standards by providing a prudent and appropriate regulatory framework.
- Providing effective stewardship over health resources by demanding accountability for achieving outcomes, including financial, managerial and clinical accountability, and by providing the frameworks, including enhanced service planning at national level, to improve the overall governance of the health system.

- Fulfilling obligations in relation to the EU, the WHO, the Council of Europe and other international bodies and the continued implementation of the cooperation agenda decided by the North/South Ministerial Council.[147]

In August 2005, Professor Brendan Drumm took up the post of chief executive officer of the HSE.[148] He stated that one of his goals was to simplify the health system so that it would be easier for people to access the services on offer. His overriding priority was the development of integrated clinical and administrative teams. He said that a specific priority was enhancing the role of nurses, including an increase in the number of clinical nurse and midwife specialists in many areas as the team-based approach was further developed. In July 2008, the HSE announced[149] that a national director of clinical care and quality is to be appointed to support greater clinical involvement (i.e. doctors, nurses, therapists, etc.) in planning and managing care services at both national and regional level.

HIQA

An important contribution to the structural reform of the health services contained in the recommendations of the *Prospectus Report* was the creation of the HIQA. In May 2005, the Minister for Health and Children established the Interim Health Information and Quality Authority (iHIQA), with responsibility for making the administrative and organisational plans for the establishment of HIQA.[150] Following the signing into law of the *Health Act, 2007*,[151] HIQA was established on a statutory basis in May 2007. HIQA is responsible for driving quality and safety in Ireland's health and social care services through:

- Setting standards in health and social services
- Monitoring health care quality
- A social services inspectorate
- Health technology assessment
- Health information.

The creation of HIQA was seen as a significant step on the road to a major improvement in the quality of health services in Ireland. Its work spans the entire health and social services system, with the exception of mental health services, which is the responsibility of the Mental Health Commission. In March 2007, a *News Update*[152] from the then iHIQA reported on the supporting role it would play in the new Commission on Patient Safety and Quality Assurance established by the Minister for Health and Children. The Commission was being asked to report to the Minister within eighteen months with proposals for greater accountability within the Irish health system in relation to patient safety, including reporting on 'adverse clinical events', a system for licensing public and private providers for health care and better integration of the work of the different regulatory bodies in the health system. The Commission on Patient Safety and Quality Assurance published its report, *Building a Culture of Patient Safety*, in August 2008. It sets out a clear and comprehensive road map for driving improvements in safety and quality across the health service.[153]

The Commission follows on from the publication of the report[154] on the findings of Professor Des O'Neill, a consultant gerontologist, on the problems at Leas Cross Nursing Home, which brought the question of patient safety very sharply into the public domain. A practical example of how this is already happening is provided in a report in the *Irish Times* of a case where a woman's diagnosis of breast cancer was delayed by eighteen months because of test errors at University College Hospital Galway:[155] an independent review of pathology services at the Galway hospital was commissioned and subsequently conducted by the HIQA.

NHS Reforms

The audit of structures and systems undertaken by the Prospectus team revealed that the system was no longer suitable for the provision of a fully accountable, efficient and effective health service in the twenty-first century, and its recommendations, along with those of the other elements of the reform programme, heralded the most comprehensive reform of the health services ever conducted in Ireland. Much of what is happening now, as part of the Health Service Reform Programme in Ireland, is very similar to the developments that have taken place in Britain in the NHS over the past twenty years. The 1980s saw central government make a concerted effort to achieve greater managerial control over the NHS.[156] The major changes during the 1980s were due to the Griffiths-inspired reforms in 1985, which were based on the finding that the NHS had no coherent system of management at a local level.[157] The reforms introduced included:

- A rejection of the 'consensus' style of management by the introduction of general managers in health authorities, hospitals and units. This was done with the intention of strengthening strategic management and accountability by putting in place structures for line management and devolved budgets.
- Policy and strategy were separated from management within the NHS by the creation of the health service supervisory board (responsible for strategic direction) and the NHS management board (responsible for management, performance reviews of regional health authorities and finance).
- Management budgets were introduced into hospitals.
- Information on clinical activity, finance, estate management, staffing and support services was generated, based on the introduction of a package of national performance indicators.
- The NHS Training Authority was established to improve management training and education.

In 1989, the British Government produced a white paper, *Working for Patients*[158] that led to:

- An increased emphasis on the separation of policy and executive/management functions with the creation of the NHS policy board and the NHS management executive.
- The removal of representatives of the health professions and of local authorities from the boards of the health authorities, which were now made to resemble company boards, composed of senior executives and non-executive directors.
- Increased power for local managers in the negotiation of contracts with consultants and in the performance management of consultants.

During the early 1990s, the British Government also introduced the GP contract, performance-related pay and a patients' charter.[159] Overall, there was a greater emphasis on consumer choice and improvements in quality of service. The *National*

Health Service Community Care Act, 1990[160] provided for the creation of an internal market within the health services by separating the financing and purchasing of care from the provision of care. It also provided for the creation of self-governing NHS Trusts for the provision of services (acute hospitals, mental health services and ambulance services). GPs with large practices (initially set at 11,000 patients and later reduced to 5,000) were allowed to apply to become fundholders.[161]

There was a gradual move away from the internal market approach, fuelled by evidence that it did not increase consumer choice. Policy emphasis subsequently shifted towards the health of the population and giving greater priority to primary care, which is very similar to what is happening in the HSE today, in particular through the HSE's transformation programme.

From 1999 on, the NHS experienced a substantial increase in funding under the Labour Government. This was accompanied by what has become known as the modernisation agenda,[162] based on *The NHS Plan: A Plan for Investment, A Plan for Reform*.[163] The plan provided for a major increase in spending, accompanied by a multi-themed agenda of modernisation, including greater patient and public involvement; opening up the NHS to alternative providers; new frameworks for raising performance, standards of care and levels of accountability; training and development for staff; and shifting power closer to the front line. All of this was supported by the development and implementation of a comprehensive new human resources (HR) strategy and an increased emphasis on the use of technology and multidisciplinary working.

In April 1998, the rolling programme of national service frameworks (NSFs) was launched. The NSFs are long-term strategies for improving specific areas of care that set measurable goals within set time-frames. The NSFs were introduced in *A First Class Service: Quality in the New NHS*.[164] The NHS plan emphasised the role of NSFs as drivers in delivering the modernisation agenda. National clinical directors were appointed as experts responsible for the implementation of a designated NSF. Examples of designated areas include coronary heart disease, mental health, diabetes, cancer and older people. Each NSF is delivered with the assistance of an external reference group (ERG), which brings together health professionals, service users and carers, health service managers, partner agencies and other advocates. The ERGs are similar to the expert advisory groups (EAGs) set up by the HSE as part of its transformation programme.

Policy and Executive Functions

In Ireland the separation of policy and executive function represents a fundamental change in the role of the Department of Health and Children. A speech[165] by Michael Scanlan, secretary general at the Department of Health and Children, delivered at the annual conference of the National Council in November 2006, outlined some of the implications of this change in role. He emphasised that policy is ultimately a matter for the Minister, Government or Oireachtas, as appropriate. The civil service provided policy advice to Ministers and Government but decisions on policy were ultimately a matter for the political system. The role of the Department, therefore, was an advisory one in relation to policy formulation. In the development of this policy, he said, the Department cannot make policy in an ivory tower: it cannot be separated from service delivery.

Secretary General Scanlan stated that one of the core messages of the *Prospectus Report* and the *Brennan Report* was that the HSE should focus primarily on service delivery and the Department should have the primary role in policy. He said that in practice, however, the Department and the HSE needed to work closely together to test the practicality of policy proposals and to listen if the HSE identified possible policy gaps, to seek greater clarity in policy objectives or to suggest that some aspects of policy needed to be changed to meet broader policy objectives. Some of this, he added, could be achieved through the work of the EAGs created by the HSE. He said that the overall aim was to protect the right and obligation of the Minister to make policy and to avoid being parochial or defensive about how policy was formulated.

HSE Transformation Programme

In December 2006, the HSE launched the *Transformation Programme 2007–2010*.[166] The programme followed consultation with staff during 2006 and reflects the views expressed during a series of meetings and events across the organisation. It also reflects the views gathered from engagements with the board of the HSE. The transformation programme states that the purpose of the HSE is to enable people to live healthier and more fulfilled lives. The programme is intended to provide employees of the HSE with a shared direction and focus that will enable them to achieve their ambitions for the future, which is that everybody should have easy access to high-quality care and services in which they have confidence and which staff are proud to provide. In a message in *Health Matters*, the HSE's newsletter, in summer 2006,[167] the CEO stated that services must reach out to patients, enfold them, and keep them out of acute hospitals and as close to their own homes as possible. At the same time, he said, the local and acute service should be linked together to ensure that patients, GPs, therapists, specialised nurses, advanced paramedics and other health professionals have ready access to specialised expertise on a twenty-four-hour day, seven-days-a-week basis. The theme of the transformation programme, therefore, is integration of services across the primary–acute care continuum.

In 2007, the HSE, as part of the programme, commissioned a detailed review[168] of acute hospital bed utilisation in hospitals throughout the country with an emergency department. The aim of the review was to assess the extent to which patients occupying adult medical and surgical acute beds had been inappropriately admitted to those beds, and the extent to which patients occupying adult medical and surgical acute beds could have been treated in a more appropriate setting, and identification of those more appropriate settings. The review identifies some implications for the role of nurses and midwives in the increased provision of community-based and home-based care across all settings. These include improved access to generalist, specialist and advanced practice nursing and midwife services (in general, psychiatric, intellectual disability and children's nursing and midwifery). There will be a need to increase resources in the community to support the provision of improved access to home care packages, intravenous therapy in the home, and community nursing to support self-care. Other implications include enhancing the role of nurses and midwives in implementing protocol-led discharge, and early involvement of community-based nurses and midwives in the planning of patient discharge and transition to non-acute care. There is also a need for the role of the nurse and midwife to focus on health promotion, particularly in relation to diet, physical activity, smoking, alcohol, substance abuse and prevention of illness.

The conclusions and recommendations of the review report confirm the HSE's vision of pressing ahead with a policy of integration of community-based care and acute care and shifting resources into the community rather than providing more beds in the acute services. The recommendations include:

- Increasing provision of a broad spectrum of community-based and home-based care to reduce admissions, facilitate timely discharge and ensure convenient, patient-centred care
- Increasing access to diagnostics and assessment without admission
- Increasing the range of non-acute bed-based alternatives available
- Implementing protocol-based discharge planning and use of estimated dates of discharge
- Reviewing internal hospital processes to reduce patient delay.

The review was conducted in thirty-seven hospitals across the eight hospital networks between November 2006 and February 2007 (excluding the Christmas period), and 3,035 patients were randomly sampled out of a population of 8,322 (36 per cent).

Evidence of practical moves towards the integration of primary and acute services was provided by the HSE's review of health services in the north-east,[169] which was conducted in 2006 by an independent group of consultants charged with developing an action plan for improving safety and achieving better standards for health services in the north-east. According to a report in the *Irish Times*,[170] the transformation of services in the north-east is to be broadened and accelerated. Up to forty primary care teams (PCTs) are to be developed in the north-east as part of the reconfiguration of primary, community and continuing care services. This amounts to an integration of hospital and community services and is intended to act as a blueprint that can be rolled out in other parts of the country.

It was reported in *Health Matters*[171] that an extensive mapping exercise of existing services was being undertaken to support service reconfiguration. This was to facilitate the rollout of 500 PCTs and 130 social care networks throughout the country. In defining the criteria for the establishment of a PCT, the HSE stated that core minimum team members would include GPs, practice nurses, occupational therapists, PHNs, physiotherapists, speech and language therapists, social workers and home helps. Extended team members, who will be called upon as required, will include specialists in dietetics, orthodontics and dental. Each PCT will be part of a primary and social care network, which will link three to five teams with responsibility for the community-based health care needs of populations from 30,000 to 50,000 people.

In response to concerns about the lack of integration within the HSE and the establishment of separate pillars for the NHO and the PCCC, Professor Drumm was reported in the *Irish Times Health Supplement*,[172] on the occasion of the roll-out and acceleration of the review and integration of services in the north-east, as saying that there would be a significant reconfiguration within the HSE's PCCC services, which, he said, was essential for the effective reconfiguration of hospital services.

Further evidence of integration of services is the hospital in the home (HITH) initiative, launched by the HSE in March 2007,[173] which allows suitable patients to be treated at home rather than in a hospital. The initiative is available to all patients currently attending the six acute hospitals in Dublin, which include the five teaching hospitals (Dublin academic teaching hospitals – DATHs) and Connolly Hospital in Blanchardstown. Potential users can also be referred through their GP if they are within the Dublin city and county catchment area, or may be transferred to the programme from a hospital or ward once they have stabilised sufficiently. This reduces the risk of patients catching hospital-acquired infections, reduces queues and reduces treatment time. According to the *Irish Times*, it was estimated that since its establishment over 1,400 bed days had been saved.

Community intervention teams (CITs) were introduced as pilot initiatives in a number of locations throughout the country (two in Dublin and one each in Cork and Limerick) in 2006. This is essentially an 'out of hours' nursing service, delivering nursing care in the home, or at a designated wound clinic. The aim is to support people at home, either allowing them to be safely discharged from hospital or to prevent them from needing admission to hospital in the first place. Patients who have been referred to a CIT are managed for a maximum of ten days and are then referred to the PHN service. Those patients eligible to use this service include older people living alone, people who have had a fall with subsequent fracture, or those who need nursing assistance to administer insulin. Types of nursing care provided include blood pressure monitoring, wound dressings (excluding compression dressings), palliative care, diabetic care, catheter care, ostomy care, percutaneous endoscopic gastronomy (PEG) tube care, respiratory care, medication management, care of Hickman catheter and peripherally inserted central catheter (PICC) lines, fractures and injections.

There is also evidence of a move towards more midwife-led services, involving an enhanced role for the midwife in the community, e.g. through the DOMINO initiative, which involves closer links between the hospital and the community. In 2007, the HSE commissioned a review of maternity services that is expected to provide a clear direction for the strategy of maternity services for the next ten years.[174]

ICT has emerged as an important area for developing quality integrated systems within the health services that are transparent, accountable and responsive to patient needs. Some progress has been made along these lines with the establishment in 2003 of Healthlink Online, which was expanded in 2006 to include a neurology service called Neurolink. Healthlink provides details of a patient's emergency department attendance, waiting list notification, radiology results, discharge information and outpatient appointments. The *Irish Times Health Supplement*[175] reported that over one thousand GPs were registered to the service along with the five DATHs; the Children's University Hospital, Temple Street; University College Hospital Galway; Mayo General Hospital; Limerick Regional Hospital; and Midlands Regional Hospital. The service was expanded in December 2006, in conjunction with St Vincent's University Hospital, to include Neurolink, an electronic referral system that enables GPs to consult with a neurologist for advice on what tests a patient with a neurological complaint may need. The HSE is also rolling out a laboratory test request service for Healthlink Online, which handled more than two million messages in 2007.

The potential for ICT uses within the health services goes beyond the administrative side of quality and safety into what is referred to now as e-health. There are developments in the diagnostics, treatment and monitoring of health care services that are being driven by the possibilities presented by modern technology. This includes the possibility to monitor large complex intensive care units with fewer personnel and to provide remote services to patients. This impacts on both the economics of health care delivery and on maintaining a patient-centred approach.

With the increasing use of remote diagnostics, remote consultation, electronic health records and more technology-assisted monitoring, the profile of the kind of health care professional that is required will change appreciably. This requires much reflection and consideration about the future. The implications go beyond the realm of the professionals and affect the way in which stakeholders conceive of and design the health care environment of the future. An interesting example of how this is being applied to the development of nursing and midwifery is what is known as the technology informatics guiding education reform initiative (TIGER).[176] This United States initiative is aimed at enabling practising nurses and midwives to fully engage in what the authors refer to as 'the unfolding digital era of health care'.

As part of its transformation programme, the HSE has set up a number of expert advisory groups (EAGs) as an integral part of the HSE's quality strategy. They provide a platform for health professionals and service users to participate actively in the programme by influencing and setting operational policy, strategy and quality standards. Participants in the groups include medical consultants, doctors, nurses, therapists, carers, managers, people who use the services, leaders in health and social care, and representatives of the Department of Health and Children. To date, groups have been set up in mental health, diabetes, children and elder care.[177]

As part of the overall reform of structures within the health services, it is possible to identify a move towards increased provision of services by the private sector, with significant political backing for this trend. Public sector hospitals are increasingly using private service providers, and the National

Treatment Purchase Fund (NTPF) is a good example. Established in April 2002, the NTPF is one of the initiatives outlined in the health strategy to reduce long-term waiting lists. The NTPF sources treatment for qualifying patients in hospitals in Ireland, Northern Ireland and England. Patients who opt for treatment with the NTPF will receive their treatment free of charge. If a public patient is on a public hospital in-patient waiting list for more than three months, he or she can contact the NTPF to discuss options for treatment in a private hospital. Medical consultants are now adapting their service provision strategies to take account of this. The NTPF has fundamentally changed the way in which hospitals deal with waiting list issues and has taken away the pressure that existed around the management of waiting lists.

Other Reports

A number of other strategies and reports have been published that are of direct relevance to nurses and midwives in the development of their roles. They include:

- The cardiovascular strategy, *Building Healthier Hearts*[178]
- *Ireland's Changing Heart: Second Report on Implementation of the Cardiovascular Health Strategy*[179]
- The *National Health Promotion Strategy*[180]
- *Report of the National Advisory Committee on Palliative Care*[181]
- The national drugs strategy, *Building on Experience*[182]
- The primary care strategy, *Primary Care: A New Direction*[183]
- *The Years Ahead: A Policy for the Elderly*.[184]

These documents refer to the role of nurses and midwives in the education of patients and clients and in promoting a positive approach to health. They also provide the basis for the development of specialist roles in areas such as cardiovascular care, palliative care and work with drug abusers and cover the role of the nurse and midwife in both primary and acute settings.

Conclusions

It is possible to identify a number of key conclusions from this review about what health services of the future will be like in

Ireland, over and above those already identified in the conclusions to Chapter 3.

These can be summarised in the following points:

- The health services of the future will be delivered by an integrated accountable entity. It will lead to a greater degree of accountability within the system. The creation of the HSE should lead to greater equality of access to services and to the development of higher standards in the delivery of services. The HSE is likely to face pressure for increased integration of services and administrative structures and, in particular, to revise the division between the two pillars, PCCC and NHO. The structures, as they are currently configured, are more suitable for bureaucratic control and distribution of funding resources than for service delivery management. They are also not conducive to the clinical management of services. (In July 2008, the HSE announced, as part of plans to speed up service integration, that the NHO and PCCC will come under the leadership of a single national director of integrated service delivery.)[185]
- In order to make progress in the integration of services, there is a need to review the involvement of clinical leaders at all levels of the health service delivery structures. This may require the creation of posts at national and regional levels for clinical coordination, involving hospitals and primary care teams. The involvement of clinicians and the integration of services are essential to ensure clinical safety throughout all of the activities of the HSE. (As noted, the HSE announced in July 2008 that a national director of clinical care and quality is to be appointed to support greater clinical involvement (i.e. doctors, nurses, therapists, etc.) in planning and managing care services at both national and regional level.) A clustering system may be appropriate with a view to bringing together primary care and hospital structures within regional and local geographic areas.
- The creation of the HSE has significant implications for the role of the Department of Health and Children. Its role changes from one of resource management to one that focuses on policy, protection of the public and performance management. This will require the development of

procedures and protocols to ensure that clinical safety is an integral part of the policymaking and performance management process. This has implications for the culture and day-to-day work of those who work in the Department of Health and Children and for the relationships that should exist between the Department and the HSE.

- The health services of the future will see acute hospitals focus entirely on major acute interventions. Service delivery will shift to the primary care setting in the community, with an increase in initiatives such as the hospital in the home (HITH) and community intervention teams (CIT). There will be an increase in the availability of diagnostic and assessment services that do not require admission to hospitals. Length of stay in hospital will be shorter and there will be more protocol-based early discharge arrangements in place. Professionals will follow up with the patient in the community.
- There will be an increase in the provision of private health services. Consumers will be offered and will avail of greater choice.
- HIQA and the respective regulatory bodies of the different professions will drive standards in both private and public health care provision. This will mean a significant increase in the quantity and intensity of audit within the system, with consequences for the way professionals account for their work. The health services of the future will be delivered with a very high emphasis on personal and professional accountability within the system. This has implications for managers and clinical professionals within the system, who will expect to be accountable for their area of service delivery and be called to account for the quality and value for money of the services they provide.
- The services of the future will be driven by a greater and more widespread use of technology, in particular information and communications technology. This will lead to an increase in the level of technology-driven services, the availability of e-health options and the networking of professionals and systems across institutional boundaries. It will underpin the increased emphasis on community-based services and remote consultation.

CHAPTER 5

Two Key Issues in Strategic Planning

Recruitment and retention are the principal challenges facing the professions of nursing and midwifery. Ireland is not unique in this regard as similar situations pertain in other countries. The work of the Commission on Nursing revealed that nursing and midwifery in Ireland suffered from problems arising from disempowerment and lack of leadership. The Commission saw these problems as contributing significantly to the slow pace of development of the professions in the past. In response, important policy initiatives have been put in place that are relevant to the future development of the professions. The need for a strategic response to the future developmental needs of the professions is also not unique to Ireland. There are many examples of good practice in this area in other countries - the United States and the United Kingdom in particular - and in international organisations. An examination of some of these experiences will furnish lessons that need to be borne in mind in formulating a strategy for the professional development of nursing and midwifery in Ireland.

Recruitment and Retention

Concerns about the recruitment and retention of nurses and midwives in Ireland over recent years have prompted a number of initiatives aimed at understanding the issues better and devising strategies to deal with them. In 2002, the Department of Health and Children commissioned a detailed study, *Towards Workforce Planning*[186] that for the first time took a comprehensive approach to workforce planning for nursing and midwifery. One of the major outcomes of the report was the establishment of the national nursing and midwifery human resource minimum dataset for use by all organisations employing nurses and midwives.

The *Towards Workforce Planning* study described the dataset as a critical instrument for the successful implementation of workforce planning and recommended that it be adopted and used by all organisations employing nurses and midwives, stating that it was essential that information on turnover rates and vacant posts should continue to be collected and the underlying reasons for leaving employment should be analysed. The report recommended that the NMPDUs should collect and collate this data on a regional basis and submit it for national collation and analysis. There is evidence that the NMPDUs are doing this. However, there is a need to address the question of continued national collation and analysis, as there is no evidence that this is being done at the time of writing.

A related study,[187] also published by the Department in 2002, indicated that turnover in nursing and midwifery varied enormously throughout the health system. Across hospital bands and services, the overall turnover rate had decreased from 17 per cent in 1999 to 15 per cent in 2000 and to 14 per cent in 2001. While turnover rates was not at levels experienced in other countries, it was a pressing issue requiring focused attention. Factors affecting turnover, as revealed by the study, included issues such as age, work experience, tenure, kinship responsibilities, education, promotional opportunities, pay, distributive justice, work environment, alternative employment opportunities/job market, job commitment, job satisfaction and behavioural intention.

In 1999, the nursing recruitment and retention group published[188] the outcome of an analysis of vacancies in the hospitals that formed part of the group. The group recommended a number of initiatives that were intended to contribute to an improvement in the attractiveness of nursing and midwifery for recruitment purposes and an improvement in the working conditions of those already in the professions. These initiatives were in the areas of continuing professional development, induction programmes, improvement of contracts, introduction of more flexibility in working hours, return to work initiatives, provision of crèches and increased participation in work committees.

Other countries have taken special initiatives aimed at retaining nurses. In the United States, the American Academy of Nursing reported on hospitals that were able to recruit and retain highly qualified nurses in a competitive market. These were known as the Magnet hospitals. Research showed that hospitals that met the criteria for accreditation as Magnet hospitals by the American Nurses Credentialing Center had better outcomes than non-Magnet hospitals.[189] The principal feature of Magnet hospitals is a focus on creating job satisfaction opportunities for nurses by creating professional nursing practice opportunities.[190] Magnet hospitals embody a set of organisational attributes that nurses find desirable and that create a work environment more conducive to the provision of nursing care. This was seen as having a significant impact on recruitment and retention of nurses.

A Department of Health and Children report in 2001[191] recommended the introduction of the grade of health care assistant/maternity health care assistant as a member of the health care team to support the nursing and midwifery function. It was intended that the introduction of support workers should allow nurses and midwives to spend more time engaged in direct patient care. The report also recommended that appropriate provisions be made for the education and training of these support workers. As a result of the recommendations of the report, a national pilot programme for the education of health care assistants was introduced in 2001. This consisted of a Level 2 training programme, developed specifically for health care assistants by FETAC (NCVA) (Further Education and Training Awards Council (National Council for Vocational Awards)) in conjunction with key stakeholders. On conclusion of the course, participants were awarded a FETAC Level 2 health care support certificate. In 2002, an evaluation of the national pilot programme for the education of health care assistants was carried out[192] and the main recommendation was that, due to the success of the health care support certificate, it should be delivered again and should be developed and expanded to train all health care assistants across Ireland.

Additional initiatives in the training of support staff include the SKILL (securing knowledge intra lifelong learning) project,[193] which was set up as a partnership between the trade unions and the HSE to provide education, training and development opportunities to staff working in support grades within the Irish health and personal social services. The project provides education, training and development initiatives to around 28,500 support staff and support service managers in the health services, including health care assistants, porters, catering assistants, household staff, semi-skilled persons/craftsperson's mates, maintenance persons, home support workers, community carers, family support workers, general assistants, therapy assistants, speech and language assistants, laboratory aides and laundry staff.

In May 2007, the HSE and the SKILL project team commissioned a national review of the role of health care assistants in Ireland, to establish their role and function in the HSE on completion of the health care support programme (FETAC Level 5). A report is in preparation. Two years earlier the skills and labour market research unit (SLMRU) in FÁS had published a health care skills monitoring report as part of a series of monitoring reviews on the supply and demand of skills in different economic sectors in Ireland.[194] The 2005 report had set out to identify current and future shortages of health care skills and to suggest approaches to tackling any gaps that may exist between supply and demand. It identified three groups of occupations, each of which displayed different supply demand characteristics and required different approaches:

- **Group 1** consisted of occupations for which an increase in training places, as well as a continued focus on appropriate human resource strategies, was the most appropriate response to the gap between projected domestic supply and demand. The report stated that these occupations had long-term supply shortfalls, which could not entirely be filled by other means (registered children's nurses were included in this group). It further stated that increasing training places for these occupations in isolation would not be the best policy. Other methods of eliminating shortages included adjusting the skills mix between the occupations, improving retention rates, promoting immigration and increasing productivity. The report concluded that, in the short to medium term, immigration would continue to play a key role in filling positions in these occupations. Once graduates from new or expanded courses begin to enter the workforce, the need for immigrant workers would be reduced.
- **Group 2** consisted of occupations where there was a possible shortfall of domestic supply in the future. Increasing

domestic supply by increasing training places might be an appropriate response in the medium term, depending on how the demand situation developed. However, other methods of reducing shortages should be introduced and evaluated before additional training places were considered. The nursing occupations in this group included registered general nurses and health care assistants. The report recommended a continuance of the current policies and an assessment of their impact before increasing training places. Current policies include adjusting the skills mix between occupations, improving retention rates, promoting immigration and increasing productivity.

- **Group 3** consisted of occupations where there was no major gap between domestic supply and demand. The nursing occupations in this group include registered intellectual disability nurses, registered public health nurses, registered psychiatric nurses and registered midwives. For these occupations, the report forecast that there would be no immediate shortages of supply up to the year 2014 but that the situation should be closely monitored.

In order to address the problems of recruitment and retention of nurses and midwives, therefore, it is necessary to develop strategies that are based on accurate statistics that monitor trends and provide a solid basis for forecasting supply and demand patterns in critical areas. It is also necessary to address workplace issues that determine the attractiveness of the work of a nurse and midwife for potential recruits and for existing professional staff.

Empowerment and Leadership

The *Report of the Commission on Nursing* identified a number of perceptions that related directly to management and leadership within the professions. These were:

- A need for greater internal communication within organisations
- That nurses and midwives, and nursing and midwifery, were not sufficiently involved in strategic planning or in policy and strategy development
- A lack of partnership and consultation between general management and nursing and midwifery management and

between nursing/midwifery management and nurses/midwives in setting and attaining corporate goals
- That nursing and midwifery management were preoccupied with hierarchies and the detailed control of nurses and midwives rather than the management of the nursing and midwifery functions.

The report identified a need to examine the recruitment, selection and training of nurse/midwife managers in order to ensure that the professions would have an effective cohort of leaders capable of responding to changing service needs. It also advocated greater devolution of authority within the nursing and midwifery management structures. These issues were also identified in a supplementary report prepared for the Commission on Nursing: *Management in the Health Services: The Role of the Nurse.*[195] Responding to this, the Commission made specific recommendations regarding internal communications within health service organisations, professional and personal career planning and the involvement of nurses and midwives in the strategic planning of the nursing and midwifery services. It also made recommendations regarding the roles of nurses and midwives in the management of their professions and their involvement in general management and emphasised leadership in both general management and clinical settings.

The Department of Health and Children subsequently established the institutional structures recommended by the Commission, and also set up a high-level steering group on the empowerment of nurses and midwives. In September 2003, the Department issued the final report of the steering group, entitled *Nurses' and Midwives' Understanding and Experiences of Empowerment in Ireland.*[196] The principal findings and recommendations for action contained in the report are summarised in Table 3.

Finding 5 of the study (see Table 3) refers to the report produced by the OHM,[197] on nursing management competencies, which identified a number of key competencies required for each of the different levels of nursing management:

- At the **top level**, these included strategic and system thinking, establishing policy, systems and structures, leading

Table 3: Empowerment of Nurses and Midwives in Ireland

Findings of the Research	Recommendations for Action
Organisational Development	
1. Nurses are invisible in organisations – they are not involved in organisational decision-making and they lack information about their organisations	• Review organisational communication strategies in order to tackle the issue of invisibility • Ensure balance between medical, nursing/ midwifery and administration input to strategic planning and decision-making
2. Nurses perceive a lack of recognition and reward for innovation in practice	• Establish and implement best practice in areas of enabling, recognising and rewarding effective innovation in clinical practice
3. Staff shortages are a barrier to the provision of quality nursing care and to enabling access to continuing education	• Implement effective workforce planning to meet existing and future HR and service needs • Link performance feedback and objective setting to objectives and strategic needs of organisation • Implement action plan recommended by nursing and midwifery resource group
Management Development	
4. Management style is an important influence on empowerment	• Adopt a systematic approach to the identification of nursing and administrative training and development needs • Deliver appropriate training and development programmes to meet those needs
5. Nursing management is influential in enabling clinical staff to function in an empowered manner	• Provide ongoing appraisal and support to nurse managers across the health service • Make wider use of the nurse management competencies framework
Practice Development	
6. Nurse-/midwife-led practice is an empowering and enabling innovation	• Build on existing initiatives to further enable innovation in nurse-/midwife-led services and extend these practice models across all nursing and midwifery divisions and areas of practice • Provide appropriate support for education, research and pilot projects • Nurses and midwives must themselves seize the opportunities offered by these developments
7. Personal and professional confidence is central to empowerment	• Explore, identify and implement interventions aimed at fostering the professional and personal confidence and self-esteem of nurses and midwives

Table 3: (*Continued*)

Findings of the Research	Recommendations for Action
8. Difficulties accessing resources needed for client needs, particularly in the area of intellectual disabilities	• Review and develop systems to ensure appropriate access to the resources required to meet client needs, particularly in the area of intellectual disabilities
9. Difficulties in meeting increased public expectations and demand for health services created by publications into which nurses and midwives have had no input	• Provide nurses and midwives with appropriate preparation in order to enable them to deal effectively with increased public expectation and demand • Ensure clinical nursing/midwifery input into the development of health service information material aimed at the general public, especially those publications dealing with health service provision and consumer rights
Education	
10. Adequate education and continuing education are critical to empowerment. Barriers to accessing education include staff shortages, with nurses and midwives having to find their own replacement cover, geographical distances and lack of resources for staff development and training	• Safeguard access to appropriate continuing education by identifying and meeting resource (both human and financial) and geographical requirements • Provide for e-learning opportunities, aimed at increased effectiveness and optimising use of resources • Provide a greater emphasis on the use of informal, on-the-job training, recognising that much of nurse and midwife learning takes place in the clinical setting • Make greater use of personal development plans • Explore other mechanisms to deliver training: coaching, mentoring (internal and external), action learning and clinical supervision • Centres of nurse education potentially have a primary role to play in promoting the professional development of all staff. Their evolving role should assist in meeting needs identified in the report
11. Concerns and uncertainties about scope of practice, accountability and legal issues	• Provide continuing and accessible education about the scope of practice and practitioner accountability within the evolving legal framework in which nursing operates

on vision and values, stepping up to the corporate agenda and adopting a development approach to staff.

- At **middle management level**, they included a proactive approach to planning, effective coordination of resources, an empowering/enabling leadership style, setting and monitoring performance standards and negotiation skills.
- At **front-line level**, they included planning and organisation of activities and resources, building and leading the team and leading on clinical practice and service quality.
- There were also **generic competencies** that should be present throughout nursing and midwifery. These included promoting evidence-based decision-making, building and maintaining relationships, communication and influencing relationships, service initiation and innovation, resilience and composure, integrity and ethical stance, sustained personal commitment and practitioner competence, and professional credibility.

These competencies provide a description of what empowered, confident, professional nurse/midwife managers will look like and how they will behave. The empowerment study, on the other hand, describes an institutional setting that militates against empowerment. Nurses and midwives 'feel invisible' (Table 3, finding 1), they are not communicated with and they feel a lack of recognition for their innovation and practice.

Using an expanded form of Kanter's model,[198] Laschinger[199] looked at the impact of structural and psychological empowerment on job strain in nursing. She points out that organisational restructuring in health care settings over the past decade has had profound effects on the way health care is delivered. Nurses in particular have been adversely affected by restructuring. Campbell[200] notes that cost-driven changes in management methods systematically devalue nurses' knowledge and displace their professional judgement. The same author also claims that nurses have been required to absorb a disproportionate amount of the cost containment burden and that, rather than increase productivity, these changes have resulted in patient dissatisfaction and increased work stress among nurses. Given that restructuring may endanger patient care, it is critical to find ways to help nurses to do their work effectively.

In one landmark 1994 study,[201] Aiken, Smith and Lake demonstrated that hospitals with strong supportive nursing work environments had significantly lower mortality rates than those that did not. These findings are consistent with Kanter's theory of organisational empowerment. They are also consistent with the findings of the Department of Health and Children's empowerment study, which identified staff shortages (see Table 3, finding 3) and difficulties in accessing resources (finding 8) as consequences of restructuring that disempowered nurses and midwives. The inability to access basic financial resources for practice, through a system of budget devolution and accountability, militates against any possibility of developing an empowered nursing and midwifery workforce.

Laschinger and colleagues[202] concluded that leader-empowering behaviours significantly influenced employee perceptions of formal and informal power and access to empowerment structures (information, support, resources and opportunity). Higher levels of perceived access to empowerment structures predicted lower levels of job tension and increased work effectiveness. They concluded that this empowered workforce required new models of leadership and a 'letting-go' of the control formally held by managers. In times of great organisational change, leaders needed to develop skills and attitudes that facilitated individual and organisational transitions necessary for success in redesigned empowering work settings. A later study[203] links empowerment to restructuring and re-engineering issues in organisations. It identified the need to move away from command and control to coordination, integration and facilitation. Managers have to seek ways of regaining the trust of employees as restructured nurses' work environments recover from the impacts of successive downsizing and changes.

Attempts have been made to measure staff empowerment within health service organisations. A survey was conducted of 457 hospital staff, including professional, support and administrative staff.[204] The factor analysis indicated three dimensions of empowerment: behavioural, verbal and outcome empowerment. These dimensions were positively related to leadership behaviour that encouraged self-leadership and negatively related to directive leadership. The three dimensions discriminated between the empowerment level of managers compared to that of non-management staff. Empowerment predicted organisational citizenship behaviour and job behaviours related to quality improvement. Klakovich[205] looked at scales of empowerment through the development and psychometric evaluation of the reciprocal empowerment scale, which was the scale used in the Department of Health and Children's empowerment study. In addition to the importance of building personal and professional confidence, this empowerment study addressed professional development with reference to nurse-led services (Table 3, finding 6), the importance of access to adequate continuing education (Table 3, finding 10), and the importance of support in addressing scope of practice issues (Table 3, finding 11).

The findings and the foregoing discussion raise the question of empowerment in the clinical environment. The work of the National Council, in developing a clinical career pathway for nurses and midwives and providing a framework within which progress can be made along this clinical career pathway, provides the basis for the development of empowered clinical professionals. This is supported at a regional level through the work of the NMPDUs. The empowerment study, however, failed to make any reference to the work of the NMPDUs or to the work of the National Council. These bodies were already operational at the time, albeit at an early stage in their development.

The National Council was responsible for the development of a clinical career pathway from generalist to specialist to advanced practice for nurses and midwives in line with the recommendation of the Commission on Nursing (see Chapter 2). This is underpinned in a number of publications:

- In 2001, the National Council published *Clinical Nurse/Midwife Specialists Intermediate Pathway*[206] and *Framework for the Establishment of Advanced Nurse Practitioner and Advanced Midwife Practitioner Posts.*[207]
- In 2002, the National Council published *Guidelines on the Development of Courses Preparing Nurses and Midwives as Clinical Nurse/Midwife Specialists and Advanced Nurse/Midwife Practitioners*[208]
- An evaluation of the role of CNS/CMS was carried out and the results were published in *An Evaluation of the Effectiveness*

of the Role of Clinical Nurse/Midwife Specialist in Ireland.[209] The results of the evaluation provided the basis for a reassessment of the framework documents
- This was followed by revised editions of the frameworks for CNS/CMS and ANP/AMP posts[210]
- In 2005, a preliminary evaluation of the role of the ANP was carried out and published as *A Preliminary Evaluation of the Role of the Advanced Nurse Practitioner.*[211]

The staff nurse, staff midwife, CNS/CMS and the ANP/AMP have a crucial role in providing clinical leadership to nurses and midwives in the clinical setting. They also have a role in providing mentoring, education, training and guidance to nurses and midwives in both the clinical and formal educational settings. Furthermore, they are instrumental in initiating and leading clinical research in nursing and midwifery. Their role therefore goes a long way towards addressing the issues raised in the empowerment study under the headings of practice development and education. The creation of these posts, in line with the provisions of the framework documents, involves consultation and cooperation between local nursing and midwifery management and the NMPDU, resulting in recommendations for inclusions of these posts in the service plan. In this way, nursing and midwifery is becoming more proactive in the shaping of health services through service planning.

The National Council was also responsible for creating new opportunities for continuing education for nurses and midwives that pre-empts the findings of the empowerment study and in particular finding 10 (Table 3). As an initial step, the National Council published *Criteria and Processes for the Allocation of Additional Funding for Continuing Education by the National Council*[212] in 2001 and an updated version in 2007.[213] This publication provided a step-by-step guide to the procedures to be followed by directors of nursing and midwifery in cooperation with the NMPDUs to access funding for continuing education programmes. As additional guidance, the National Council in 2003 published *Guidelines for Health Service Providers for the Selection of Nurses and Midwives who might Apply for Financial Support in Seeking Opportunities to Pursue Further Education.*[214] The website of the National Council also contains information for nurses and midwives on educational and development opportunities provided by third-level educational establishments. The National Council has funded continuing educational opportunities for nurses and midwives, including courses, workshops, seminars, conferences and other events.

The Department's empowerment study calls for more attention to be given to personal development plans for nurses and midwives (Table 3, finding 10). The National Council has published two editions of *Guidelines for Portfolio Development for Nurses and Midwives*,[215] both of which provide a structured framework for nurses and midwives to build their own professional development profile.

In addition to these activities and publications, the National Council has carried out a number of detailed analyses of professional development issues for nurses and midwives. These include:

- *Agenda for the Future Professional Development of Nursing and Midwifery*[216]
- *Report on the Continuing Professional Development of Staff Nurses and Midwives*[217]
- *An Evaluation of the Extent and Nature of Nurse-Led/Midwife-Led Services in Ireland*[218]
- *Clinical Nurse Specialist and Advanced Nurse Practitioner Roles in Emergency Departments: Position Paper*[219]
- *Clinical Nurse Specialist and Advanced Nurse Practitioner Roles in Intellectual Disability Nursing: Position Paper 2*[220]
- *Clinical Nurse Specialist and Advanced Nurse Practitioner Roles in Older Persons Nursing: Position Paper 3*[221]
- *Service Needs Analysis for Clinical Nurse/Midwife Specialists and Advanced Nurse/Midwife Practitioners.*[222]

The empowerment study provides an in-depth analysis of nursing and midwifery in Ireland and shows a professional cohort within the health services that views itself as being disempowered. The literature review confirms that there is a need to create structures and practices within organisations that ensure the free flow of information and facilitate involvement of individual managers in decision-making as a basis for the creation of a sense of empowerment. The literature also highlights the negative impact that organisational restructuring can have on nursing and midwifery, which is of particular relevance in Ireland as the Health Service Reform Programme is implemented.

Much progress has been made in Ireland through the work of the National Council and the NMPDUs, in close cooperation with the directors of nursing and midwifery, to create the conditions necessary for the emergence of empowered, fully professional nurses and midwives. Much of this progress has been made in the period since the publication of the empowerment study, from 2001 to the present. The research undertaken for this book (Chapters 8, 9 and 10) seeks to throw light on how far nursing and midwifery has come and how much remains to be done as a basis for the formulation of a strategy for the development of the professions in a changed health service. If nurses and midwives are to become more empowered within the health services, leadership must come from within the professions.

There is a close link between empowerment and leadership. Kanter, in the classic book *Men and Women of the Corporation*[223] maintains that work environments that provide access to information, resources, support and the opportunity to learn and develop are empowering. In such an environment, employees are encouraged by management to act on their expertise and judgement and, accordingly, they are able to accomplish their work successfully. As a consequence of empowerment, employees are more committed to the organisation, have higher levels of trust in management, are more accountable for their work and are less likely to experience job strain. Empowerment therefore must be seen as a condition that is necessary for the emergence of leaders within organisations.

A study[224] of nurse leaders' perceptions of what comprises successful leadership in today's acute inpatient environment set out to gain understanding of their perceptions of both the value of their roles in today's health care settings and their beliefs about how power and gender interface with role worth. The study referred frequently to Kanter's structural theory of organisational behaviour. Sixteen nurse leaders were recruited for the study in seven Magnet and nine non-Magnet hospitals. The results of the deductive analysis supported Kanter's theory: 83 per cent of nurse leaders confirmed that access to power, opportunity, information and resources created an empowered environment, producing a climate that fostered leadership success and enhanced levels of job satisfaction among nurses.

One Irish researcher, Dr Marie Carney,[225] has looked at middle manager involvement in strategy development in not-for-profit organisations in Ireland and, in particular, the director of nursing's perspective. She also looked at how organisational structure impacts on the role. Her study detailed the problems experienced by directors of nursing within organisations: exclusion from strategic decision-making resulting in poor communication flow and lack of access to senior managers, resulting, in turn, in a sense of isolation, of being controlled and of decisions being made that were of major concern to nursing and the organisation without any involvement from the director of nursing. Carney highlighted the critical role directors of nursing should have in nursing management and the wider health service context.

Nursing and nurse management have enormous potential to influence health care strategy and health care delivery. However, in order to do this, it will be necessary to work in multidisciplinary cooperation and alliance-based models of care delivery. Nurses will have to demonstrate strategy development and planning and the delivery of effective evidence-based and efficient nursing care and be seen to benefit the health service as a whole. This involves a fundamental reappraisal of the role of the director of nursing, including shedding of non-strategic elements of the role and the empowering of clinical nurse managers. It involves, therefore, the creation of an organisational environment in which leadership emerges as a result of empowerment.

Writing in the context of the NHS in the United Kingdom,[226] Fradd identified the following competencies and attributes that were needed to lead within a political environment:

- Political astuteness
- Compassion
- Ability to work independently
- Being an effective collaborator
- Ability to develop high trust relationships
- Self-confidence tempered with humility
- Respect for the process of change as well as the content
- Ability to work across business functions and units.

Fradd concluded that, in the case of directors of nursing, the lack of an appropriate balance between the strategic role, leading nursing and being responsible for operational matters has not infrequently left them isolated and the target of blame. It has been suggested by Sofarelli[227] that transformational leadership approaches will assist nursing to develop into an empowered profession, with the potential to be a dominant voice in reshaping the health care system of the future, especially during periods of uncertainty arising from significant organisational and structural reform (as is the case in Ireland at present). Because of the inherent uncertainty of health care, leadership requires individuals who are capable of making decisions, with a committed, long-term vision of what can be accomplished, capable of identifying common values with staff needs.

A review of the literature on leadership, in Ireland and other countries, shows a number of common themes and it is possible to identify three critical levels on which leaders operate and which demonstrate three families of competencies and skills.

First, leaders are individuals who have a clear set of values, which they are capable of converting into a vision of what they want, and can articulate this vision lucidly. It is this combination of values, vision and ability to articulate that sets leaders apart from others. It includes the ability to distinguish between the operational demands of a role and the need for a strategic approach to development. It implies that leaders do not become lost in operational detail. It also implies that leaders are reflective thinkers, with a defined philosophy based on values. In this way, leaders create meaning and provide opportunities for people to learn.

Second, leaders are also individuals who are good at building relations with others. As managers, they empower those around them and motivate them to high standards of performance and achievement. The capacity to relate, empower and motivate is thus a key competence in a leader. It includes skills such as the ability to read the environment, particularly the political and policy environment, and the possession of a high degree of political astuteness. It also includes the ability to cooperate and collaborate across the organisation, across the professional disciplines and across organisational boundaries.

Leaders are people who inspire trust and confidence in those with whom they come in contact and they manage the use of power within organisations in a way that engenders this trust. In this capacity they act as process consultants, bringing together different aspects of the organisation towards the achievement of the vision. It involves, therefore, a multidisciplinary approach that is non-hierarchical and that respects the contribution of each discipline to the achievement of the overall vision. Relationship building also entails the development of mentoring and support mechanisms aimed at addressing issues of succession and the emergence of future leaders.

Third, leaders are individuals who plan their way forward and are capable of operationalising their vision in a manner that focuses on achievements and results. Leaders are results-focused and outcomes-oriented. This includes a deep understanding of the business side of organisations and the importance of harnessing all of the business disciplines towards the achievement of the vision. It also includes the ability to work in an independent and accountable manner. This implies that nurse leaders need to broaden their skills and educational base to include experience and training in disciplines that are not part of the clinical set of skills for nurses. It also involves linking individuals and their skills sets with the appropriate tasks that need to be done. Planning also entails the provision of arrangements capable of preparing future leaders and ensuring that they receive the necessary mentoring and support. This kind of leadership is usually referred to as transformational or symbolic leadership because it works on the basis of empowering others and distinguishes itself from transactional or management leadership, which is more focused on the management of processes and procedures.

In order to encourage the emergence of such leaders, however, organisations need to create an environment within which these competencies can flourish. Figure 1 summarises the key competencies and levels of activity involved in leadership that are of relevance to nursing and midwifery in Ireland.

A leader is someone who is in possession of a system of values that forms the basis for the articulation of a vision. A leader also possesses an active network of relations within and outside the organisation and, through the articulation of the vision, empowers and motivates those around him or her. The system of relations and networks provides the structures within which a

Figure 1: Values, Competencies and Activities Relevant to Leadership in Nursing and Midwifery

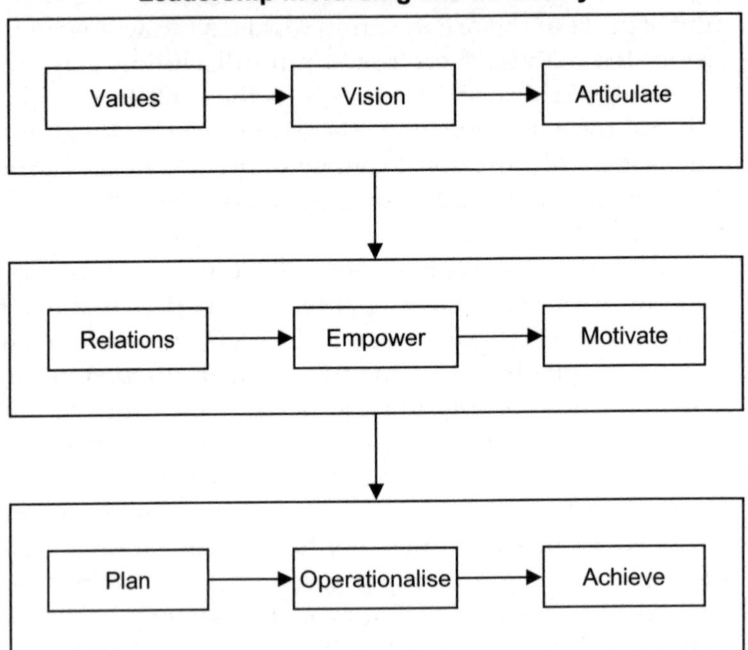

plan can be conceived, operationalised and delivered. This model of leadership is driven by vision, with empowerment at its centre, and is focused on achievements.

To summarise on the overall issue of leadership and empowerment, the work of the Commission on Nursing has had a profound impact on nursing and midwifery in Ireland. Through the implementation of its recommendations, conditions for the professions now exist in Ireland to develop in a way that would not have been thought possible before. In particular, the creation of the nursing policy division within the Department of Health and Children, the National Council and the NMPDUs means that the professions are well positioned to develop in a proactive way that influences the development of policy and matches the needs of the services and of the professions.

The transformation of educational provision at pre- and post-registration levels opens up new possibilities. The introduction of the pre-registration degree programme looks set to change forever the way in which nurses and midwives view themselves and the way in which they interact with other professionals within the health services. Nursing and midwifery now have a clinical career pathway that works in favour of retaining the experience and talent of expert nurses in the clinical area. There are also opportunities for a more integrated approach to be taken between the services, the third-level institutions and the professions for the development of joint appointments. In short, nursing and midwifery seem well positioned to advance confidently into the future as key players in shaping and moulding the provision of health services in Ireland.

Despite the progress made to date, research such as the empowerment study indicates that nurses and midwives still feel disempowered within the health services. They perceive themselves as invisible within the system when it comes to taking the real decisions and they are not involved in shaping policies or service delivery mechanisms. There is a crisis of identity within nursing and midwifery that is militating against the emergence of leadership. It is also calling out for the emergence of leaders who are capable of articulating the values of the professions and providing a vision for the future. There is a need also for leaders who are capable of building meaningful relationships across all of the services and are able to motivate and empower nurses and midwives in the fulfilment of their role. These leaders need to be at the centre of the strategic planning of nursing and midwifery services and to convert plans into activities that meet the needs of the services.

When set against the major changes that are taking place within the health services as a result of the Health Service Reform Programme, and taking into account the significant changes introduced as a result of the recommendations of the Commission on Nursing, it is clear that we are living through very turbulent times for the health services in Ireland, and for nursing and midwifery, as key players within those services. This is likely to be a reality for the foreseeable future. Many positive things are happening and have happened, but there is still evidence of a lack of fit between the changes being introduced and the positioning of the professions of nursing and midwifery within the services.

CHAPTER 6

Learning from International Strategies for Nursing and Midwifery

A number of strategies for the development of nursing and midwifery have been developed in recent years outside Ireland. A brief review of strategies developed by the WHO, as well as strategies in the United Kingdom and Canada, is highly relevant in developing a strategy for nursing and midwifery in Ireland.

WHO

In 1993, the WHO produced a report, *Nursing in Action: Strengthening Nursing and Midwifery to Support Health for All.*[228] This was the culmination of the work of a group of experts throughout Europe who set out to build on the decision taken by participants at a 1988 WHO European conference on nursing and to choose the strategy of health for all as the guiding star for the development of the profession. They set themselves the goal of creating a new kind of nurse who would be an autonomous, skilled practitioner who could work alone or in partnership with other professionals to deliver primary health care in any setting. The role would not be to serve another profession but to inform, support and care for the patient and the community. The report contained advice and guidance that could assist nurses throughout Europe in developing this role by creating the necessary support structures, establishing regulatory systems, reforming education, preparing leaders and managing change. It is a guide to practice and professional development.

It identified four major functions that are at the core of nursing:

1. Providing and managing nursing care, which includes actions that are promotive, preventive, curative, rehabilitative and supportive, to individuals, families or groups.

This is most effective when it follows the logical steps inherent in the nursing process
2. Teaching patients or clients and health care personnel
3. Acting as an effective member of a health care team
4. Developing nursing practice through critical thinking and research.

It was based on an understanding of the implications of these core functions that strategies and approaches to education, regulation, practice development and professional development should be developed.

In 1995, a WHO expert committee on nursing practice[229] met in Geneva to define strategies for change to ensure that nursing practice, consistent with the principles of primary health care, were developed with the genuine participation of the community. To achieve this, the committee set out to describe the core elements of nursing practice; to specify the nature and scope of nursing practice in countries at different stages of socioeconomic development; to identify the implications for and action needed with regard to basic nursing education, continuing nursing education, management of health services, legislation and regulation, working conditions and research; and to consider the implications for and action needed with regard to the development of health services and human resources. The committee reviewed the definition of what nursing is and made a series of recommendations for the WHO and for the member states of the WHO.

For member states, the committee recommended, in particular, that strategies should be developed to enable nursing and midwifery personnel to provide comprehensive and integrated primary, secondary and tertiary health care. The committee endorsed the recommendations contained in the report of a WHO study group, *Nursing Beyond the Year 2000*,[230] which had made a series of recommendations to the WHO and its member states. The recommendations were intended to promote within member states a new multi-sectoral systems approach to health care delivery and full collaboration of health care personnel at all levels; a shift in the focus of the workforce development in nursing and midwifery to reflect country health needs, with particular emphasis on vulnerable groups; and a revitalisation and reorientation of nursing and midwifery education and practice to meet the challenges of the future.

Among the recommendations, the group highlighted that an important dimension of strategic planning for nursing and midwifery was the creation of a multi-sectoral forum of relevant partners involved in practice, research, education, management and policy development for nursing and midwifery services, in order to address the changing needs of nursing and midwifery personnel, their preparation and the development of educational systems that would allow personnel to move from one career level to another. It also recommended flexible and enabling regulation and legislation and the creation of a variety of educational and career pathways for nurses and midwives.

In 1999, the WHO produced a strategy[231] in response to what was perceived as the increasing complexity of the environment in which nursing and midwifery had to operate. It set out a number of principles that should guide the development of nursing and midwifery education and also provided guidance for the development of a curriculum. Among its recommendations was a list of supporting subjects that should be included, as a minimum, in the curriculum, making explicit their application to nursing and midwifery. These included:

- Public health, health promotion, health education and therapeutic patient education
- Social and behavioural sciences
- Biological sciences
- Research awareness
- Communication
- Professional, ethical and legal issues
- Information management and information technology
- Management, leadership and organisation.

In 2002, in response to growing shortages of nursing and midwifery personnel in member states, the WHO published *Nursing Midwifery Services: Strategic Directions 2002–2008*.[232] This was intended as a framework for collaborative action to support countries in enhancing the capacity of nursing and midwifery services to contribute to national health goals. The document identified five key result areas, each with specific objectives and expected results. These were:

1. **Health planning, advocacy and political commitment**: National development and health plans provide for adequate nursing and midwifery services and expertise.
2. **Management of health personnel for nursing and midwifery services**: National employment policies are implemented for the nursing and midwifery workforce that are gender sensitive, based on healthy and safe work environments and conditions, provide for equitable rewards and recognition of competencies, and are linked to a transparent career structure.
3. **Practice and health system management**: Nursing and midwifery expertise is fully integrated into decision-making processes at all levels, and health systems use best available practices for the care of individuals, families and communities.
4. **Education of health personnel for nursing and midwifery services**: Competent practitioners with an appropriate skill mix are available to deal effectively with the current and future challenges of practice.
5. **Stewardship and governance**: Stewardship and governance of nursing and midwifery services involve the Government, civil society and the professions to ensure the quality of care.

England

In 1999, the Department of Health outlined the British Government's strategic intentions for nursing, midwifery and health visiting,[233] and described a number of measures to be taken by the Government to strengthen the role and contribution of the professions to the delivery of health care. The strategy contained a number of what it described as 'early milestones' to measure progress. These included the improvement of pay and conditions for nurses, midwives and health visitors, more nurses, midwives and health visitors, more training places, and professional development initiatives. Among the latter were:

- Guidance about the establishment of nurse, midwife and health visitor consultant posts

- Exploring the benefits of clinical practice benchmarking with the nursing, midwifery and health visiting professions
- Taking forward nurse prescribing
- Publishing plans to show how nurses, midwives and health visitors would have access to programmes to strengthen leadership and management across the NHS
- Beginning the process of preparing for new legislation for professional self-regulation
- Implementing a programme to develop the public health aspects of nursing, midwifery and health visiting
- Working with women, midwives and others to explore opportunities for an expanded midwifery role
- Publishing plans for the better management of NHS-funded education in which the Department of Health would take on a more active and wider role
- Producing a strategy to influence the research and development agenda, strengthen the capacity to undertake nursing, midwifery and health visiting research, and use research to support practice
- Preparing personal development plans for nurses, midwives and health visitors
- Developing a new model of nurse education
- Establishing a partners' council to explore and make recommendations about the potential for greater standardisation of roles and titles
- Partners' council to advise on pre- and post-registration education.

Scotland

The Scottish Executive Health Department produced a strategy for nursing and midwifery in Scotland in 2001.[234] This proposed a number of key drivers for the strategy. These were:

- Accountability, support and supervision
- Leadership
- Professional development
- Career development and workforce planning
- Research, evidence-based practice development and innovation
- Education.

The key action points were identified as follows:

- Supporting children and families through a network of carers and professionals
- Supporting people with learning disabilities
- Supporting older people
- Defining competencies in forensic nursing
- Working to promote social justice in communities
- Supporting patients in the community
- Supporting nurses in remote and rural areas
- Improving services for patients with chronic disease
- Assessing the impact of nurse and midwife consultants
- Setting new standards in A&E (accident and emergency) nursing
- Piloting the family health nursing role
- Developing nurse prescribing roles
- Monitoring role expansion
- Enhancing professional accountability
- Developing clinical supervision
- Building networks for isolated practitioners
- Supporting newly qualified nurses and midwives
- Improving supervision for midwives
- Training, supporting and supervising support workers
- Developing leaders in nursing and midwifery
- Recognising the significance of ward sisters/charge nurses
- Enhancing professional development
- Developing competency-based frameworks
- Creating options for student nurses
- Expanding career pathways
- Addressing issues in workforce planning
- Promoting research, evidence-based practice, development and innovation
- Addressing issues in nurse and midwifery education.

Wales

In 1999, the National Assembly for Wales published a strategic framework document for nursing, midwifery and health visiting.[235] It stated that the strategic goal for the professions was to realise the full potential of nursing, midwifery and health visiting in order to meet, in collaboration with others, the future health needs of people in Wales. It identified five supporting aims that would help achieve the strategic goal. These were:

1. **Improving the environment of care**: To ensure that nurses, midwives and health visitors coordinate the environment of care for their patients and clients, thereby ensuring, through collaboration with others, that all appropriate resources were centred on the patient/client.
2. **Ensuring high-quality service for all**: To ensure that high-quality nursing, midwifery and health visiting care reached all those in need, whether rich or poor, wherever they may be, to promote good health, and to prevent, cure or relieve suffering, with the patient/client as an equal partner in care.
3. **Encouraging independent and reflective practice**: To ensure that all nurses, midwives and health visitors developed their practice in a reflective and evidence-based manner, founded upon a standard of education that enabled them to practice as equal partners with other health care professionals, supported by continuing professional development and clinical supervision.
4. **Developing existing and new career paths**: To develop existing and new career paths for nurses, midwives and health visitors which allowed senior staff to remain clinically involved if they so wished, and which would break down unhelpful barriers between education, research and practice, as well as between nursing, midwifery and health visiting and the wider health care context.
5. **Demonstrating the value of nurses, midwives and health visitors**: To demonstrate the value of nursing, midwifery and health visiting so that the professions, together with colleagues and the service as a whole, appreciated the particular contribution which the professions make to the health of patients and clients.

Northern Ireland

In 2003, the Department of Health, Social Services and Public Safety (DHSSPS) of Northern Ireland published its strategy for nursing, midwifery and health visiting,[236] which reviewed the achievements in implementing a strategy that had been developed in 1998, with actions in six areas: commissioning, practice, education, research and development, leadership, and management. The DHSSPS has also prepared jointly with the Department of Health and Children in Dublin a number of papers[237] on the contribution of nursing to public health that attempted to identify on an all-island basis strategies for improving the contribution of nursing and midwifery to public health. In addition, the DHSSPS has published a strategy document[238] that provided a strategic framework for the health services and for the development of health care professions into the future.

United Kingdom

In 2005, the four United Kingdom chief nursing officers (CNOs) established the modernising nursing careers initiative. A UK-wide group of nursing leaders formed the Modernising Nursing Careers Board, chaired by the CNO of England. Their report contained a description of what modern careers in nursing should be like.[239] The characteristics they identified included:

- An up-to-date picture of nursing careers characterised by opportunity and diversity
- Care taking place in and outside hospital with the workforce moving between them and nurses starting their career in the community
- A career framework that allows nursing to 'grow its own' with multiple entry points for those taking up nursing as a second career or as mature entrants
- Plurality of provision offering alternative employers and employment models including NHS Foundation Trusts, self-employment and social enterprises
- A flexible principle-based curriculum built around patient pathways, with a strong academic foundation and interdisciplinary learning
- A framework that supports movement between career pathways, practice, management and education and that values and rewards different career types
- Better balance of generalists and specialists to provide integrated networks of urgent, specialist and continuing care

- Careers built around patient pathways using competence as the currency for greater movement and flexibility
- A career structure with an increased number of assistants working as part of multidisciplinary teams
- Standardisation of advanced level skills
- Patient pathway-based careers focusing on nursing roles rather than titles
- Nursing roles defined according to patient need – to provide intervention that is timely, accurate and swift
- Nursing teams more self-directed and professionally accountable
- Nurses leading, coordinating and commissioning care, as well as giving care, to bring about change measured by health gain and health outcomes
- Care based on evidence and critical thinking and assisted by new technology.

Canada

The first nationwide nursing strategy for Canada was developed in 2000 as a response to a severe shortage of nursing personnel.[240] In 2005, a pan-Canadian steering committee consisting of representations from the various branches of the nursing profession, employers, unions, educators, physicians and provincial and territorial governments produced a final report on the first phase of a project for nursing human resources.[241] The goal was to ensure an adequate supply of skilled and knowledgeable nurses to meet the evolving and changing health care needs of all Canadians. The report recognised that health system restructuring over the previous ten years had had a negative impact on nurses, resulting in significant changes in the nursing workforce.

According to the report, health care organisations had struggled to cope with health reform, fiscal challenges and changes in the nursing workforce by implementing policies that had had a negative impact on the quality of work-life of professional nurses. This included, for example, increased involuntary and unpaid overtime for nurses, casualisation of the nursing workforce, increased use of unregulated health care providers and increases in workloads. These developments had resulted in a growing dissatisfaction among professional nurses and many had chosen to leave the profession. The report also stated that it was now recognised that these changes in the professional work life of nurses were having a detrimental impact on the quality of patient care. The report made recommendations to address the priorities, based on three broad categories of health human resources: health human resources planning; retention and recruitment; and inter-professional education for collaborative patient-centred practice.

Lessons Learned

There are a number of important lessons that can be drawn from this brief review of strategies for nursing and midwifery from outside Ireland. These are:

- The importance of a coordinated approach at a national level to planning for the future of nursing and midwifery emerged from all of the strategic documents reviewed. Regardless of the nature of the political and administrative system within a country, planning for nursing and midwifery is a national priority. In Ireland, the research undertaken for this book has highlighted the lack of coordination and communication that exists within nursing and midwifery. This points to the need for the creation of a partnership forum, a strategic coordination committee at national level that includes all the key stakeholders for nursing and midwifery and encourages an integrated approach throughout the professions at local and regional levels.
- There is a need for rolling strategic planning in nursing and midwifery at national level. This should be based on a clear understanding of the way in which the environment is evolving, a vision of what is required, a clear set of objectives, targets with timeframes for delivery and clear allocation of responsibilities for delivery. When formulating strategies, the views and needs of all stakeholders should be included and time should be allowed in order to reflect changing needs. Strategic planning needs to be future-focused and based on an analysis of trends in society and in service development and a description of the likely shape of the health services of

the future. It should also focus on the competencies that will be needed to address the future needs.

- Nurses and midwives need to be involved at every level of the planning and development of policies and delivery mechanisms, at national, regional and local levels and need, therefore, to develop the competencies required to contribute at this level.
- Nursing and midwifery need to develop a strong sense of professional identity as a basis for nurse-/midwife-led, autonomous services related to patient/client needs and service development priorities. The professions should work as integrated partners with other professionals and health care workers, participating as members and, where appropriate, as leaders of these teams. But the professions should also create their own specific range of services in response to the changing needs of the professional environment. Interdisciplinary, interprofessional, multidisciplinary approaches to education, professional development, service planning and delivery should be second nature to nurses and midwives, rooted in a strong sense of their own professional identity and the contribution they make to health care. Nursing and midwifery need to organise themselves for the delivery of services in a manner that takes full account of the efficiency and effectiveness that can be achieved through the application of good skill mix practices, involving professional and non-professional staff. Good teams are built on the principle of complementary skills and roles.
- The roles of nursing and midwifery are evolving in a dynamic way in response to increased complexity in the environment (political, administrative, financial, technological and cultural). This has implications for the way in which nurses and midwives are educated for entry to the professions and for the ongoing professional development support they need to fulfil their role. Curricula for nurse education at pre- and post-registration levels need to reflect this. Nurses and midwives require broad-based education aimed at developing competencies that evolve in line with the needs of the service. Nursing as a science is based on research, evidence-based practice, specific knowledge and skills, whereas nursing as an art is based on intellectual and

emotional competencies that form the basis of reflective practice and the development of wisdom and judgement. Nursing practice needs to expand its boundaries, based on clear guidance on scope of practice and on the basis of competency frameworks, supported by adequate education and professional development.

- There is a need for a balanced approach to specialisation within nursing and midwifery. The important role of the generalist nurse or midwife must be maintained, as the principal coordinator of care in a health care setting. This must be based on a rich career pathway that covers clinical, management, education and research opportunities. Career pathways should be integrated to enable flexible movement between and within the pathways, encouraging linkages and close relationships between all of the pathways.
- Nursing and midwifery must have strong roots in the community. Primary care is increasingly becoming the principal forum for the delivery of nursing and midwifery services where they can be close to the homes of patients and clients and strengthen their presence by providing a unique set of services that are tailored to the needs of patients and clients.
- Planning for an adequate workforce in nursing and midwifery requires information systems at a national level that permit the creation of strategies for recruitment and retention based on workforce planning. This includes planning the environments in which nurses and midwives work in a manner that takes account of the need for safety and encourages nurses and midwives to achieve their full potential. Planning for nursing and midwifery resources needs also to take account of the importance of flexible, gender-sensitive policies. Planning of this kind is particularly important at times of health service reform to ensure that undue stress is not put on the nursing and midwifery workforce.

PART 2

Researching Key Stakeholders and Opinion Influencers

Chapter 7

Key Stakeholders and Opinion Influencers

This research is the most comprehensive survey of key stakeholders and decision influencers within the Irish health care services ever conducted, with 115 individuals participating in one-to-one personal interviews or in focus groups. The aim of the research was to identify future roles for nursing and midwifery within the Irish health services from the perspective of key stakeholders within the services, and to identify the professional development implications for this role. The research was undertaken for the purpose of making a major contribution to the creation of a professional development strategy for nursing and midwifery in Ireland that would reflect and adapt to the likely pace of change within the health services and was capable of addressing the needs of the professions.

The research was broken down into thirteen objectives. These were to:

1. Identify and analyse the contexts (policy, economic, organisational and institutional) within which the health services of the future will be delivered
2. Describe the likely future shape of the Irish health services
3. Describe as clearly as possible the new role that is intended for nurses and midwives within the services
4. Describe in what way this role differs from the current role
5. Assess the degree of clarity, certainty and understanding, or otherwise, that exists in relation to the definition of this role among key stakeholders
6. Describe the nature of the relationships that will need to be developed within new institutional and service delivery settings
7. Identify the skills and competencies that will be required to fulfil the new role

8. Assess whether these skills and competencies differ from those that are currently required
9. Assess perceptions as to whether nurses and midwives currently possess the necessary skills and competencies
10. Assess the level of preparedness of nurses and midwives to work within the dynamics of the new relationship and contexts
11. Assess the adequacy of the current provision of professional development opportunities for nurses and midwives (at pre-registration and post-registration levels) to prepare them for the challenges inherent in the new role that is envisaged for them
12. Identify what changes would be required to the provision of professional development opportunities to ensure that in the future nurses and midwives are adequately prepared for their role
13. Formulate a professional development strategy for nursing and midwifery adapted to the likely pace of change within the health services and capable of addressing the needs of the professions.

Before commencing the study it was necessary to identify the key stakeholders in the Irish health services, in terms of those whose position and opinions would bear directly on nursing and midwifery. After a detailed review, the following categories were selected for research:

1. Policymakers
2. Service managers
3. Medical consultants
4. Educators
5. Directors of the NMPDUs
6. Directors of nursing and midwifery (hospital and community)
7. Regulators of nursing and midwifery.

The members of these categories of stakeholders are the main drivers of national strategy for nursing and midwifery. Other important categories include:

8. Assistant directors of nursing/midwifery
9. Clinical nurse managers/clinical midwife managers (CNMs/CMMs) – grades 1, 2 and 3 (see Appendix 5, point 4)

10. Specialist nurses and midwives (including CNSs/CMSs and ANPs/AMPs)
11. Staff nurses and midwives.

The eight principal groups were broken down further:

1. **Policymakers** – It was possible to identify a core group of individuals in key posts within the Department of Health and Children who were involved in determining the shape of health services in the future and the role of nursing within those services. These were:

   - Secretary general
   - Assistant secretary responsible for strategy implementation
   - Head of project strategy implementation
   - Director of personnel section
   - Chief nursing officer
   - Chief medical officer
   - Principal officer responsible for nursing policy division
   - Chief pharmacist
   - Principal officer responsible for National Task Force on Medical Staffing.

2. **Service managers** – This category can be divided into two sub-groups:

   - Group 1 – Individuals with overall accountability for the implementation of policy, the reform of the services and the delivery of services:

     - Chief executive of HSE
     - Head of change management team within HSE
     - Two members of the board of HSE
     - National directors of HSE's National Hospitals' Office (NHO), primary community and continuing care (PCCC) and human resources
     - Director of health boards' executive (HeBE)
     - Health board chief executives
     - Chief executives of major academic teaching hospitals
     - Directors of public health.

   - Group 2 – A wider group of service managers with responsibility for the delivery of services in specific geographic areas and care settings, including representatives of acute and primary care settings where there is a significant nursing component.

3. **Medical consultants** – The research concentrated on those consultants who were members of the National Taskforce on Medical Staffing and in clinical areas with nursing relevance. In addition, other medical consultants in disciplines of great relevance to nursing – maternity, gerontology and emergency – were interviewed.
4. **NMPDUs** – There are eight directors of these units in the country. All were included in the research.
5. **Educators** – It is possible to divide this category into three, each of which has historically developed in very different ways and reflects a different culture and professional emphasis:

   - Group 1 – Professors of nursing and/or midwifery and heads of schools of nursing and midwifery in universities. This group is not alone responsible for the delivery of essential services in the areas of pre-registration education, post-registration academic education and CPD, but they are also expected to take a lead in the promotion and development of research in nursing and midwifery.
   - Group 2 – Heads of schools of nursing in the institutes of technology, where the emphasis is on the delivery of pre- and post-registration educational services.
   - Group 3 – Directors of the newly formed centres of nurse education, located in the major teaching hospitals and with a specific role in the area of CPD and development of links between education and clinical practice.

6. **Regulatory Bodies** – This category covers the regulatory bodies for medicine and for nursing.
7. **Directors of Nursing and Midwifery** – There are 302 directors of nursing and midwifery (hospital and community) in the Irish health services.
8. **Trade Unions** – During the period of the research there was a great deal of industrial relations unrest within nursing and midwifery that culminated in an industrial dispute commencing on 2 April 2007 and lasting seven weeks. The

public discussions that took place at the time highlighted the important role that trade unions played in the professions of nursing and midwifery. It became apparent that trade unions were an important factor and were, therefore, included as an eighth category as part of the research.

A total of seventy-seven representatives of all eight categories were interviewed face-to-face (see Table 4).In addition, two focus groups were held for directors of nursing and midwifery in Band 1 and 2 hospitals, with a total of eleven participants; two focus groups were held for directors of nursing and midwifery in Bands 3 and 4, with a total of eleven participants; and two focus groups for directors of public health, with a total of eight participants - for a total of thirty directors of nursing and midwifery (see Table 5). Directors of centres of nurse and/or midwife education were interviewed in two focus groups in different locations and at different times (see Table 5). In all, there were thirty-nine focus group participants.

Table 4: Numbers Participating in Interviews

Category	Interviews
Policymakers	10
Service managers	35
Medical consultants	10
NMPDUs	8
Educators	10
Regulatory bodies	2
Trade unions	2
Total	77

Table 5: Numbers Participating in Focus Groups

Category	Participants
Directors of nursing and midwifery	30
Directors of centres of nurse education	9
Total	39

The ethics committee of the Faculty of Health Sciences, Trinity College, Dublin, granted approval for the research, and the standards required by the committee were incorporated into the design of the methodology.

The comments used in Chapters 8, 9 and 10 are taken from the interviews and focus group meetings and the interviewee's group is identified for each quote. All comments were made by individual participants and are not intended to be indicative of the opinions or representative of that individual's group unless otherwise apparent. In transcribing the quotes from oral to written format, some have been revised slightly for clarity.

CHAPTER 8

Research Results: The Future of Health Services in Ireland

The context in which the health services in Ireland have developed and changed has been well documented, and it is possible with the benefit of hindsight to describe this context and its impact on the present shape of these services with some certainty. The future is less certain, but the comments of informed and interested parties can form the basis on which build a realistic depiction of the health services of the future. Accordingly, the responses of all interviewees to the following two questions were probed in detail in order to obtain further insights:

- What do you think will be the major contextual changes for the health services of the future?
- How would you describe the most likely future shape of the Irish health services?

Eight main themes were used to guide the discussion around these questions:

1. A different health care consumer
2. Changing lifestyle and society
3. Separation of policy and executive functions
4. Organisational structures
5. Systems pressure
6. Accountability and value for money
7. Expectations of quality
8. The cultural challenge.

These eight themes provide a framework within which to consider and discuss the results of the research.

A Different Health Care Consumer

There was unanimous agreement among those interviewed that socioeconomic change was a significant factor affecting the future development of the health services. A feature of the feedback from interviewees was the degree of awareness they demonstrated about socioeconomic issues in Ireland today and the consistency of opinion across all the categories of issues discussed. The most frequent topic commented on was the public's increasing expectations regarding the quality and quantum of services provided (see Table 6).

Table 6: Research Issues: Socioeconomic Changes

Theme	Frequency of mention
The public will have increased levels of expectation regarding the quality and quantity of services provided	26
Future health services will be delivered in a society where increased wealth is the norm. Public expectations will increasingly establish a correlation between health and wealth	11

A recurring theme throughout the interviews and focus groups was the extent of change that had taken place within Irish society in recent years. Consumers were seen to be more informed, more discerning and more demanding, with a high level of awareness of what constitutes value for money. One policymaker made the following comment:

> We have very astute and smart consumers out there now who really know the difference between a poor quality service and a good quality service and know when they are getting value for money and when they are not.

Irish society has also changed in that there is much greater wealth available within the country. Wealth brings with it the expectation that things can be bought: Irish people expect to get more of what they want, sooner, and are intolerant of circumstances where they do not get what they expect or want. As one medical consultant said:

> We are a much wealthier country. We have raised the bar of expectation hugely and we are utterly intolerant of not getting what we want immediately, if not yesterday.

The changes in standards of living in Ireland is something that is frequently commented upon by those who have a memory of 'what things were like in the past' and is also noticed by people 'who were not living here in the past', as one educator commented. It was seen by interviewees as likely to have an impact on future health service provision. Future health services will be delivered in a society where increased wealth is the norm. Public expectations will increasingly establish a correlation between health and wealth. As a result, people will tend to be intolerant of excessive queuing and having to wait for services. One service manager put it: 'There won't be a tolerance for queues. The country is too rich and people too rich; with so much money, they would demand an alternative'. This is likely to contribute towards the possibility of alternative sources of service provision being expected (e.g. private health services).

Medical consultants, in particular, commented on their perception of the way in which consumers of health services have changed and how the increase in wealth has contributed to an increase in levels of expectation regarding the quality and quantity of services being provided. This changes the nature of the relationship between consumers and service providers. Medical consultants commented on how a more informed, wealthier client will have a different attitude towards medical consultants. Whereas, in the past, there may have been a perception that medical consultants wielded enormous power within the system, it is likely that a more informed consumer with more choices will be more discerning and look for consultants with the best skills for the service required:

> Medical consultant: People are going to come to us for our knowledge and our skills. They are not going to come for our power anymore.

Finally, the expectations of the public regarding the quantity and quality of service provision will also place considerable pressure on service providers to supply a new kind of leadership. A service manager noted that managing expectations in the light of increased costs of service provision, particularly the mounting costs of acute service provision, would require a new style of leadership.

Changing Lifestyle and Society

The themes most often stated about the likely effect of demographic and epidemiological changes on the health services are given in Table 7. Most comments referred to the multi-ethnic nature of Irish society and to issues of lifestyle-related changes that would impact on future health services.

Table 7: Research Issues: Demographic and Lifestyle Changes

Theme	Frequency of mention
Future health services will have to contend with the fact that our population will live longer and the population will be made up of more elderly people who will require more services	10
Future health services will have to contend with changes in the structure and nature of family life	11
Future health services will have to contend with changes in lifestyle, and lifestyle-related illnesses will become more prevalent	18
The multi-ethnic nature of Irish society will provide a significant change of context for future health services	30

Interviewees frequently referred to what they termed the ageing of the population. In general, it was felt that this, and the related issue of increased longevity, would be of growing importance in the years to come. One service manager commented:

> Of course, demography influences our epidemiology. The fact that we have people living longer means that the issue of co-morbidity is a major one for the future.

Ageing is seen as just one element of the significant demographic changes that are taking place within Irish society, which the interviewees acknowledged would bring new challenges for nursing and midwifery. Interviewees spoke about their concerns about the 'huge growth in population and ageing of the population, a shift from rural to urban living and the immigration factor'. This concern about the fast growth of the population is borne out by statistics, as previously noted.

The demographic changes in society, mentioned in Chapter 3, are also seen as having a significant impact on the relationships within families. The change in the relationships between dependant people and their families has knock-on effects for the health services in general and for nursing and midwifery in particular:

> Service manager: Look at the whole area of care of the elderly, and why that has become such a huge issue in recent years. I think that one of the main reasons is that families are no longer looking after their own, their old. So everybody is clamouring for care for his or her family.

It is a broad social issue, related to the question of where people live, where they work, how long they work, and the links and relationships that exist within communities. These factors change the nature of the demands that are placed on the health services:

> Educator: And then there is the other impact, that is the impact for older people and where they live and who is going to be in proximity to them when they are older, simply because of the economic change.

This suggests a need to look again at the support that is given to families and carers in their own homes, and to take account of the changing nature of family frameworks. This will undoubtedly impact on the way in which we shape the primary care provisions of the future, the aspirations of which are frequently based on a traditional view of what the family framework is likely to be:

> Service manager: People cannot afford to provide the same family unit that they did maybe thirty years ago and some of the primary care aspirations we have are predicated on a traditional family environment.

Interviewees saw economic prosperity and increased wealth within Irish society as being a major contributor to the increase in lifestyle-related issues for the health services. Many interviewees referred to changes in epidemiology related to lifestyle, and, in particular, increases in the chronic conditions of obesity, diabetes, circulatory and cardiovascular conditions, abuse of alcohol and drugs, unhealthy eating habits, and sedentary lifestyles.

Many interviewees expected these conditions to continue to grow and referred to them as 'affluence-related' conditions. One interviewee highlighted the fact that while Ireland has, and will increasingly have, these 'affluence-related' issues, this country also continues to have problems with 'poverty-related epidemiology':

> Service manager: This gives us the worst of all worlds – not really reducing dramatically the poverty-related epidemiology and acquiring

> the worst of the affluence-related issues and I am thinking of alcohol and lifestyle-related factors and obesity and the effects from obesity.

In one instance, these lifestyle-related changes were referred to by a trade union representative as a 'selfish culture' of abuse and excess. By way of contrast, however, many interviewees recognised the positive impact that the smoking ban would have on future health services.

The challenges of a multi-cultural society featured largely in comments from interviewees. The health services need to respond to the many challenges that these changes present. Typical comments were:

> Service manager: I think we are seeing huge social changes at present in relation to the fact that we have become a more multi-cultural society with fewer carers and that is certainly evident now in care of the elderly. We don't have the extended family.

> Service manager: In the last ten years, Ireland has changed and it's going to continue to change in terms of the population base, their origins, colour and, indeed, religious beliefs – and health has to respond to those requirements.

Interviewees also commented on how maternity services have experienced an increase in the birth of non-Irish national children in recent years. Multi-ethnicity and multi-culturalism present significant communications challenges within the health services:

> Service manager: The way in which we communicate or don't communicate with people is an issue and we are now starting to develop pictograms and colours as a means of communicating with people who don't have English as their first language. But the cultural emphasis and differences need to be dealt with.

Interviewees also spoke about the need to take account of the cultural background of the people who come to work in the health services. One service manager remarked: 'If we are to bring in Spanish nurses, for example, do we need to try to have a Spanish environment in some of these hospitals, as is happening in the UK?'

The danger of introducing barriers within health service delivery is also a natural corollary of multi-cultural service deliverers and clients. Interviewees spoke about the fact that people from different cultural backgrounds who come to work in the health services in the future will have some different needs:

> Medical consultant: There are language difficulties and the danger is that a significant cohort will take up the lower-paid jobs and the more menial jobs in the health service as well as elsewhere. We will have to find a way to be able to cope with the changes that this will bring in terms of communication. I fear that it will actually bring in even more social barriers within health service delivery.

The directors of nursing and midwifery who participated in the focus groups commented on the implications of social changes, such as these for the education and preparation of nursing and midwifery staff and spoke of the need for 'having our staff trained up... to manage it'.

Many interviewees recognised significant changes in epidemiology and changes already taking place in the kinds of conditions that are being treated within the health services. An educator mentioned, by way of example, 'an increase in diseases such as AIDS, HIV and syphilis, and a recognition that Ireland still has one of the highest incidences of cancer and cardiac disease in Europe'. This also has implications for the skill sets and competencies of clinical staff involved in the health service as they will be coming across diseases and conditions that they may not have seen before, such as 'conditions that are very common in tropical Africa, for example, sickle cell [anaemia]'. In keeping with trends throughout the OECD, there is a shift towards the consideration of population health issues and interviewees also raised the need for increased awareness, education and planning in that area.

Finally, there was a very strong sense of significant change having already taken place and much more to come in the future:

> Trade union representative: There is no doubt that the culture of this country has changed significantly and that change is extremely rapid. As we move forward ten years, we will see even more changes.

Separation of Policy and Executive Functions

Interviewees were fairly evenly divided between the advantages and disadvantages of the separation of policy and executive functions (see Table 8). However, they were uncertain about the nature of the changes that were envisaged. In particular, it was not clear to them how the role of the Department of Health and Children would change and how it would develop. There was also a perceived lack of clarity about the relationship that should exist between the policymaking and the executive functions.

Table 8: Research Issues: Separation of Policy and Executive Functions

Theme	Frequency of mention
There are advantages associated with the separation of policy and executive functions	21
There are disadvantages associated with the separation of policy and executive functions	22
The separation of policy and executive functions will also be accompanied by a centralisation of executive functions in one body – the HSE	40
Future health services will be delivered in a context where the role of the Department of Health and Children will change significantly – dedicated only to policymaking	34

A number of advantages were identified in the separation of policy and executive functions. Most interviewees agreed with the following comment:

> Service manager: The changes [recommended by the *Prospectus Report*] have the potential, if they are differentiated adequately in terms of role and relationships, to create an adequate tension to ensure the aspirations of the *Quality and Fairness* strategy.

These changes include the change in role of the Department to one of policymaker and monitor of implementation and performance; the creation of 'a single unitary or perhaps centralist delivery system such as the HSE'; and the creation of the HIQA, charged with development and implementation of initiatives in the areas of quality, information and standards.

Taking the politics out of health service delivery as a result of replacing the health boards with a unitary system was also seen as positive. The centralisation of service delivery that results from the separation of policy and executive functions and the creation of a single deliverer is also seen as being of value in eliminating differences across the health services, as one of the policymakers

observed. An important corollary of the separation of policy and executive is that it should allow the Department to concentrate on the formulation of policy:

> Policymaker: From the policy point of view, from the Department point of view, it allows a very clear opportunity and very clear space and a very clear set of circumstances within which far greater thought and far more time can be given to the preparation and formulation of policy.

Many interviewees, however, expressed the view that is not possible to achieve a complete separation of policy and executive functions; they depend on each other for their effectiveness and for their meaning: 'It is very difficult to make informed policy if your finger is not very firmly on the pulse of operations'. They recognised the need for those involved in service delivery to have an input into the formulation and preparation of policy. The HSE will want and need to be involved in the formulation of policy, otherwise, commented a service manager, it would be impossible for them to 'help to resolve the problems within the health service if they have no say in policymaking'.

Separating the Department from operations has the potential to lead to what one policymaker described as 'an ivory tower type existence'. This can result in local issues and needs not being considered adequately when it comes to formulating policy. So it is necessary for the Department to retain very close links with the executive functions if it is to formulate informed policy. One interviewee perceived it as being dependent on good links between both:

> Service manager: You cannot make policy without very significant inputs from the participation of executive functions and I think that the consequence of that is that the relationship between the Department of Health and Children and the Health Service Executive is very important to the success of it, and if that relationship is not right it could create very significant problems in the system.

Of central importance was the definition of the role of the Department relative to that of the HSE. Lack of clarity in this was evident in many comments. One policymaker defined the role of the Department as follows:

> To assist the Minister in the determination and making of policy; to mobilise the resources from the Department of Finance to enable those policies to be put in place; and to put in place the regulatory and legal framework within which our health services can best work.

> And then, on behalf of the Department of Health, and on behalf of the Government, to hold the HSE and the executive arm accountable for delivery on the policy decision.

This represents a very significant change in the role of the Department and in the relationship between the Minister for Health and Children and the health services. It also represents a significant challenge for those involved in the management of the role of the Department:

> Policymaker: The system in Ireland contains an expectation that whoever happens to be Minister has responsibility. If something is going wrong, even at detailed local level, such as 'why was that patient left on a trolley for three days?', he or she expects to get an answer from officials in the Department without necessarily having to go further than that. Also, parliamentary questions, Dáil business and ministerial representation are structured on that basis.

The challenge of implementing these changes within the Department is enormous and will require a significant change in expectations, in culture and in the way business is conducted. Thus, for example, according to another policymaker:

> The political system is going to have to accept that the Department of Health and Children and officials in the Department will no longer have the level of detailed knowledge and understanding that they once had of individual services... The establishment of the Health Service Executive is partly on the understanding that accountability for delivery of services will shift from the Minister to the chief executive of the HSE and his or her board. That is a critical element of the new delivery system.

In practice, this means that, in the future, if things go wrong with cancer services or childcare services, for example, it should be the chief executive and his or her staff in the HSE who should be answerable in the first instance 'and the Minister holding them to account, as opposed to the Minister constantly being expected to stand up in the Dáil and explain why such and such a thing has gone wrong in relation to a particular hospital car park or whatever the issue happens to be'. That, the interviewee concluded, is a very significant shift in accountability and 'it brings us back to culture because the culture of the system has to accept that change in accountability and who is responsible for what'.

Generally, interviewees agreed that health service delivery arrangements to date have been overly disaggregated. A unitary service should provide more equal access and be better coordinated:

> Service manager: We are moving towards a very centralised structure and that can be very good because it can give clarity in relation to services. It can push through equal access to services. It can help in terms of coordination.

Another important stated advantage of a single delivery structure is that it will provide an opportunity for increased emphasis on accountability. This is a topic that was very prominent throughout the whole of the research. Changes in the relationship between policy and executive functions were also seen as contributing to a culture of accountability. Interviewees were also of the opinion that, as one regulator said, this would 'make all of our lives hopefully more professional and more focused on the post or the purpose that we are employed for'.

Organisational Structures

Almost half of those interviewed concentrated on defining the nature and extent of primary care services, and a substantial number focused on defining the relationships between primary and acute services. The relationship between primary services and the rest of the health services is important in seeking to understand the future of the health services and the role of nurses and midwives within it (see Table 9).

The vision for hospitals of the future is one where they will concentrate on the major acute areas of intervention, requiring

Table 9: Research Issues: Organisational Structures

Theme	Frequency of mention
There are many implications for hospitals in the new health services, including the role of independent hospitals, the amalgamation of hospitals and the use of tertiary referral hospitals	18
Future health services will require the definition of new relationships between primary and acute services	38
Future health services will need to define the nature and extent of primary care service provision	77
Service development will be an important part of changes in organisational structures in future health services	24

specialist and predominantly surgical intervention. Most other services can and should be provided in the community. A movement in this direction has obvious and serious implications for the roles of nurses and midwives. Most of their work will shift to community-based settings and they could, in fact, provide a lead role in developing a wide range of community-based services that have shifted from acute hospital settings. According to one service manager, 'there is no point in nurses and doctors being left in hospitals to the degree that they are at present. They have got to follow where the patients are'.

The same interviewee commented on a range of practical situations where this could have a significant impact: 'we have hospitals in this country where we have a hundred thousand attendances at warfarin clinics'. The interviewee spoke about the implications of 100,000 people travelling to get their treatment when they should be given their treatment at home and went on to apply the same logic to diabetes and heart conditions that can be treated at home.

A number of other interviewees also expressed the view that large acute hospital centres should 'only be dealing with complex cases and surgical patients'. Most of the services that are currently provided in hospitals can and should be moved out to the community. One service manager concluded:

> That has two major impacts: it has a huge impact on nursing in terms of not having that type of work going on within the acute hospital sector... it won't be justifiable for the cost of it to be provided there. Secondly, that provides a huge opportunity for nurses to say that they will become the group who actually, to a large degree, take a lead role in how this will be provided at a community level.

The directors of nursing and midwifery expressed the view that there was an opportunity for nursing to provide some leadership in the area of relations between primary and acute care. A typical comment was:

> Director of nursing and midwifery: If you are talking about the relationships between primary and acute services, I think that it is an essential area for the nurses to actually lead on.

There remains, however, a major challenge regarding the establishment of linkages within nursing and midwifery in primary and acute settings. One service manager referred to the importance of engaging with practice nurses in the community, who work in GP practices and who, the interviewee believed, 'are very much outside the total care loop'. The interviewee said that links between practice nurses and public health nurses were not as good as they should be and that the development of these links offered many opportunities to improve the effectiveness of care delivery in the community. A number of interviewees said that the role of GPs needed to be explored more in terms of the integration of services. One service manager commented that they should be more closely integrated into the hospitals, allowing them to run clinics within the hospitals. Other interviewees pointed to instances where good working contacts had been established with GPs in the area, particularly in midwifery and obstetrics services. Where this had happened, positive changes had followed.

Interviewees cited many examples of work that is ongoing in the area of integration of nursing services in cooperation with the HSE's NHO and PCCC, looking at processes, integrating care pathways, caring case management and looking at the role particularly of the clinical nurse specialist. In view of the move towards a more integrated approach between acute hospitals and community care, a number of interviewees expressed concern about the creation of separate pillars within the HSE for the NHO and for the PCCC. At a time when the trend in the services is towards greater integration, the structures in place at the highest level did not mirror this. Interviewees referred to the problems faced by managers of acute tertiary hospitals with no input into what happens to long-stay beds in the surrounding area. If some of those beds are closed down because of lack of staff, the manager feels the repercussions on the acute system. One service manager said that integration of service management between primary and acute care should be reflected throughout the system, at both a local community level and at the highest level within the HSE. The logical conclusion would be for a single integrated management structure, involving the merger of the NHO and PCCC.

Moving towards an integrated system also has implications for the relationships between existing hospitals within the system, and their relationships with academic institutions. One of the interviewees referred to the creation of networks:

> Service manager: Regarding changes in role, I think the ultimate aim is to have a single delivery system. There is a lot to be said for that.

> However, looking at voluntary hospitals and [the Dublin Academic Teaching Hospitals], I feel that the hospitals have to look towards being able to share their services. Inevitably there will be amalgamations and I think that is going to happen within the networks that are being formed.

The role of hospitals is closely related to the question of epidemiology and the tension that exists for hospitals between their role as a provider of services in their local community and their role as tertiary referral centres with specialities that attract referrals from all over the country:

> Service manager: One of the big issues facing hospitals... is that it is both a community hospital for a local population and a tertiary referral hospital with super-national specialties, regional specialities, etc. So there is a constant tug between the two.

Many references were made throughout the interviews to the primary care strategy and to the need to invest more in primary care. It was stated frequently that the need to invest more in this area is recognised but that there are difficult choices to be made because of the traditional approach of seeing investment in health care primarily in terms of capital expenditure on buildings and technology in acute services.

One service manager referred to the difference in the investment cycle between primary and acute services. The investment cycle in primary services can be as long as forty years – the length of time it would take for a policy such as the smoking ban to take effect and show returns within the system. On the other hand, the investment cycle in acute services is a fraction of that – the results of buying a machine can be seen almost immediately. In one service manager's view, the longer-term investment in primary care is more sustainable and better in the long run but it requires a distinctive type of leadership to resist the pressure from the professions for the short-term investment. Interviewees also referred to the need for practical investment in resources such as diagnostic equipment for primary care settings:

> Service manager: We have to look at primary care settings providing an enhanced service in certain areas and maybe they should have some sort of laboratory service and an x-ray facility available to them. I think it is essential to spend some more funding on primary care, provided it's obvious that there is a return.

Systems Pressures

Interviewees were very aware of the high level of media interest in the pressures that exist within the emergency departments in major acute hospitals. They commented on issues such as the importance of developing primary care as an important dimension in resolving the problems that exist (see Table 10). The relationship between these pressures and primary care development was evident throughout the research.

Table 10: Research Issues: Systems Pressures

Theme	Frequency of mention
Future health services will have to tackle the problem of increases in activity levels in areas such as emergency departments, an increase in the numbers of patients in both acute and community services, and a demand for an increase in the number of beds in acute services	23
Future health services are likely to include an increase in private provision of services. This may be as a result of political pressure or as a result of consumer choice and the availability of new private services	35

One service manager commented on a possible contributing factor:

> The reasons why we have such difficulties in our A&E departments is that we have such a poor primary care service and our GP services are so inadequate, certainly out of hours... so I would say that we must strive for more integrated services.

Interviewees' concerns about bed numbers generally amounted to a demand for more beds. Many suggested that the Irish health services had fewer beds per head of population than comparable economies throughout the developed world. This is closely related to the issue of bed occupancy rates. Some interviewees believed that occupancy rates within the Irish system were very high compared to Europe and that this produced considerable pressure on staff.

Interviewees also related the question of bed numbers to the pressures within the system caused by the increased numbers of patients/clients being treated. They believed that the population had increased substantially without a concomitant increase in capacity and that, in addition, said a service manager, 'the population profile has changed. There are higher dependencies and that does require an increase in beds'.

The increase in numbers of patients/clients came in for particular mention in relation to maternity services:

> Medical consultant: The biggest issue facing us at the moment is the increase in birth rates. Probably from about 1998, year-on-year, we have seen something of a 3 per cent to 5 per cent increase in this hospital.

The question of bed numbers, the appropriate use of those beds that are there, the potential for alternative ways of treating patients who are admitted to acute hospitals and the integration of community and acute services are integral parts of all of the issues raised in this section of the research. The issues are similar to those discussed under the question of organisational structures. The comments made there about the HSE's *Transformation Programme 2007–2010* and its overall policy of moving towards community-based services, integration of primary and acute services and removal from the acute services of those cases that should more appropriately be treated in the community are relevant here.

The interviewees also identified a move towards increased provision of services by the private sector and a strong perception that there is substantial political backing for this. A number of interviewees pointed out that public sector hospitals are increasingly using private service providers, and the National Treatment Purchase Fund (NTPF) was quoted as a good example of the trend towards private sector provision. A medical consultant remarked: 'the treatment purchase fund is the only [element of the] health sector that has been increased'.

Medical consultants are now adapting their service provision strategies to take account of this trend:

> Medical consultant: I think our development here will be to increase our private capacity, which we will use to provide care to public patients through the treatment purchase fund and other types of initiatives like that; we will just channel the money through a different route. But those beds will be private in the sense that they will be commercially run and privately funded and that's actually what we are looking at now.

This has fundamentally changed the way in which hospitals deal with waiting list issues. The interviewee commented that the

NTPF had taken away all the pressure that existed around the management of waiting lists 'because we don't care anymore, it's not our problem. The treatment purchase fund is responsible for our long waiters now. It's their problem'.

Service managers also expressed concern about the implications of the European Working Time Directive (EWTD) and the impact it will have on staffing numbers and roles. One said:

> We've got to look at the working time directive and how it impacts on doctors and the number of doctors that are out there and the care that nurses can give and substitution care.

Concern was also expressed about the overall numbers of staff employed in the health services:

> Medical consultant: I think that one of the biggest challenges for the HSE is in trimming down its organisational structure. For a population of four million, we are grossly top heavy in terms of organisation. You could look after a population of four million with a small health board type setting, not with all the ones we have historically taken in.

Accountability and Value for Money

There exists within the health services, based on the evidence emerging from this research, a very high level of expectation that accountability, performance management and value for money will be major issues in future health service provision. The issue of accountability was the one that attracted most comments from interviewees in the research (see Table 11). This illustrates the level of interest generated by the issue and the level of awareness among interviewees of its importance.

Interviewees frequently referred to the *Brennan Report* and the *Prospectus Report* being of great importance in drawing attention to the lack of accountability that had existed within the system to date. Similarly, frequent reference was made to the important role of HIQA in defining and setting standards, in monitoring performance and in conducting independent reviews.

Service managers within the HSE were particularly conscious of the importance of accountability and the challenge involved in driving a culture of accountability throughout the whole system:

> Service manager: The accountability issue is huge. We are as an organisation going to drive accountability every day, and at the moment

Table 11: Research Issues: Accountability and Value for Money

Theme	Frequency of mention
The CEO of the HSE is now accountable for the services – not the Minister	5
It will be necessary to ensure that accountability (including clinical accountability) exists at all levels within the organisation, from the CEO and finance director through all clinical grades and administrative grades. Clinicians cannot be allowed to opt out	135
Clinicians will be expected to become more involved in the management of the services and, as a result, will need to become more accountable for the services they provide	31
There will be an increase in the quantity and intensity of audit activity in future health services, examining issues of governance, value for money, accountability and quality	25
Performance management will become increasingly important, managing and tackling underperformance	26
There will be a significant increase in the degree of political scrutiny of expenditure in health to ensure public accountability for the investment	47
There will be a greater emphasis on the need to demonstrate value for money in the provision of services, including accounting for inputs, outputs and outcomes	116
There will be a need for more critical incident analysis with reference to the tribunals of enquiry, complaints, litigation and pressure groups, in order to ensure that lessons are being learned and changes made	15

accountability within the system is, I think, not something that we score highly on and we have got to move to a situation where, in relation to all of our processes and everybody who works within the system, there is accountability and that is going to be a complete change in culture.

Many interviewees concurred with this view and there was evidence of a high degree of expectation in relation to the role that HIQA will play in promoting and developing a greater sense of accountability within the system. Interviewees were of the view that the issue of accountability translates into taking responsibility for budgets and for delivering value for money within one's own area of responsibility. But the question of accountability goes beyond finance and budgets and requires an audit-based approach to assessing outcomes. It is not just financial accountability, according to one interviewee: 'It's accountability on the best type of treatment we give the patients and there is not enough auditing of that done, auditing to see if we have done it correctly'. This raises the question of 'personal and professional responsibility', which will include more accountability for professional and managerial performance, with standards being driven and monitored by bodies such as HIQA and the professional regulatory bodies.

There is an expectation from service managers that HIQA will drive standards and protocols in a firm and authoritative way: '[The change] will be subtle, probably driven mostly by HIQA, if it does have what I would call the wherewithal, the credibility and the authority to actually drive clinical practice, the standards and protocols'.

The nurses and midwives interviewed for the research were clear about the fact that accountability is about systems and processes involving risk management and professional responsibility as part of a multidisciplinary team. Service managers see accountability as something with a hard edge, something that will affect contracts and the way in which people work. Ultimately, accountability is about demonstrating that what staff do is useful and is value for money and, in order to do that, research tools are needed that have the capacity to capture relevant data. This is a particular challenge for nursing and midwifery.

> Regulator: I think the other challenge, to be hardnosed about it, is demonstrating that what we do is useful. We don't gather useful data against which we can measure our performance and, increasingly, I think performance assessment is going to become part of our day-to-day work.

Being held accountable is also related to the potential for litigation, which raises the need for a review and assessment of the lessons to be learned from critical incidents that occur from time to time in the public arena. Recent enquiries into problems within the health services have brought to light the importance of taking stock of what is to be learned from these incidents. Interviewees referred to a number of high profile cases that have been in the public eye (e.g. the so-called Dunne Case involving the National Maternity Hospital) and stressed the need for deeper reflection on the lessons to be learned from these cases and on the need to create more widespread awareness of these lessons.

So, to drive accountability, it is important that the system is capable of taking stock of and analysing the failures as well as best practice. This requires the development of good evaluation skills. A number of interviewees commented on the importance of evaluation, highlighting that it is something that requires more concerted development effort:

> Service manager: Probably the weakest part of our current system is the monitoring and evaluation and the feedback loop, and getting that back in so that we can measure what we do with it.

This has a very practical application to the development of programmes and initiatives in the areas of clinical services and of professional development. Interviewees expressed the view that development programmes and pilot initiatives need to be evaluated in more detail and the results of these evaluations be made available as the basis for the development of a new generation of programmes and initiatives. It was seen to be the best way to learn about what the real needs were and the most appropriate response to those needs. This finds an echo in the desire expressed by policymakers that the clinicians in management initiative[242] should continue in a revitalised and enhanced format. Interviewees expressed the view that this programme had delivered real value where it was implemented, and that it had proven its ability to adapt to local conditions and local culture.

Evaluation of programmes and initiatives is closely related to the question of performance management and value for money. One service manager, in commenting on the need for more value for money analysis, said:

> Part of the problem we have in the present system is that an awful lot of good is done and we have no way of counting it and, therefore, we have no way of proving that we are doing a lot of good.

Many interviewees referred to the fact that significant investments had been made in the system in recent years and that there was considerable pressure from within the political system to demonstrate that this money was being well spent:

> Service manager: There is a constant cry from the Government that, no matter how much money they put into the health sector, they still have problems. They speak about huge increases in expenditure over the last ten years.

The all-pervasive nature of health service provision and its impact on the population is perhaps what makes it such a live political issue and one that is likely to continue for the foreseeable future:

> Policymaker:It is probably the only business in the country that has four million customers. Every single person in the country is a customer of the health service, every person who votes, every person who pays taxes, every person who consumes the health service has an interest in it and therefore that aggregates up to a major political issue.

This opinion is also reflected in the views of service managers, particularly from the point of view of seeing a return on the huge investment that is being made in the health services, and 'a nervousness that there is significant funding going into health and it doesn't appear to be addressing the needs of the people'.

The performance of the health service relative to the investment being made is also often seen by politicians as a direct result of poor management. Policymakers spoke about the pressure they experienced from ministers and politicians about what was perceived as 'indications of poor management'.

Interviewees from the academic sector, on the other hand, pointed to the fact that the increase in expenditure in health in recent years should be set against many years of lack of investment:

> Educator: OK, there has been an exponential increase in the amount of money spent in health but that is after a long period of very little spend in health. So it is very easy for politicians to fan this type of thing and say, you know, we are giving all this money and you are paying all this money through your taxes and yet what are we getting for it?

Expectations of Quality

The issue discussed by interviewees in relation to quality in the health services was the emergence of a more patient-centred service responding to the emergence of a more sophisticated consumer, with higher expectations of quality and service in the future (see Table 12). Consumers have become very smart and astute and aware of the difference between a poor quality service and a good quality service and know when they are getting value for money and when they are not.

Table 12: Research Issues: Expectations of Quality

Theme	Frequency of mention
There will be an increased emphasis on putting the patient at the centre of service development and delivery and monitoring the patient's journey through a seamless service	58
Future health services will be delivered in a society with increased access to information, including internet-based information. This will drive expectations of quality among consumers. Information technology will increase in importance as a way of managing information within the health service	42

One policymaker commented on the fact that patients/clients frequently find out about a particular illness or condition for the first time through soap operas on television, where illness and health is treated in great detail, including well-researched and graphic depictions of signs, symptoms, diagnosis and treatments. Many interviewees referred to the wealth of information that is now available on the internet and the fact that patients/clients are increasingly approaching the services with a lot of information about their condition. This enables them to engage in a much more informed and authoritative manner with health care professionals and the health care system; they have become empowered by information.

> Policymaker: One of the things we are looking at, and it is not particular to nursing, is that the whole shift in terms of the relationship between the cared-for and the carer is around this idea of empowerment. It is happening anyway. It is happening through the access to information and so on, the educational levels at which people generally are operating. The more information we feed them the more awareness/consciousness we are generating about health issues.

This interviewee said that the concept of an 'empowered' patient/client – empowered through information and education – was something that perhaps policymakers, professionals and service managers needed to reflect more on and said that it was important to 'make sure that people can get access to information that is authoritative and that can be relied upon', and that health care professionals needed to 'adjust around the more educated consumer. Empowerment is at the centre of everything we have to do – we as policymakers, and you as professionals. Otherwise, we will continue to replicate what we have done in the past and we can only get it wrong'.

The fundamental shift in the relationship between the carer and the cared-for has enormous implications for the culture of the professions. This was articulated very strongly by some of the medical consultants. According to one:

> A culture change is where doctors say we are not God, 'we know next to nothing, a little bit more than you do and you know that now because you can get on the internet and find out and say we know bugger all about much of the drugs we are prescribing. We just cannot. We are overwhelmed. There are hundreds of them. And now you are sharing that with us so let's talk as equals'.

Availability of information, therefore, and the use of information and communications technology has already changed fundamentally the way in which health care is delivered and promises to do so even more radically in the future. On the other hand, it is important that the system has the capability to track what is being done well and build on it. This highlights the need for system-wide mechanisms and information systems capable of supporting this kind of information.

One service manager lamented the fact that, despite the increased emphasis on quality, 'we can never say that we have in place structure and mechanism of delivery and measurement both qualitatively and quantitatively of what we do'. Measuring what we do is seen as an essential ingredient in developing quality. This raises the question of research into clinical practice and the importance of building a practice-based approach to research. This requires the health services to take a hard look at the way in which education systems and practice systems are focused:

> Trade union representative: To what extent are our education systems, our research systems and our practice systems capable of absorbing all of the knowledge? We have been very poor in doing it so far. For example, I am not aware of any system in this that is geared towards taking in best practice from different parts of the world, piloting it and then moving on and mainstreaming it.

Many of the interviewees mentioned the growing importance of IT skills and IT systems within the services:

> Service manager: The health service of the future is going to be an IT-enabled service and everyone who works in it is going to be working as much in a virtual way as in a natural way.

This interviewee described the potential afforded by technology for online checking of results from laboratory tests, radiology tests, and the value and safety of relying more on electronic records rather than paper records, and referred to the much-publicised example of a Cavan hospital where the death of a child, whose file could not be found, gave rise to an enquiry about the safety of paper records. Similarly, the use of bar codes and computerised order entry forms could all contribute towards the integration of the services and improved links between primary and acute services.

The service manager saw the need for shared information between professionals within a system where the client owns the information:

> So I think that we are going to have to move into the modern world where health professionals share information and that the information belongs to the patient and we get away from these professional empires where doctors don't authorise nurses, and nurses don't authorise others. All of it is creating huge risks for patients.

The directors of nursing and midwifery who participated in the focus groups referred to expectations among the public about the potential impact of technology on health service provision. They spoke of major issues of public expectation around the use of technology within the health services that need to be identified and addressed.

One policymaker referred to 'the revolution that is taking place in the linkage of ICT to health technologies and it is nothing short of a revolution in e-health that is happening'. The interviewee concluded that it was likely that these developments would impact in a very significant way on the health services in Ireland, including the way we conceive of and design the health care environment of the future.

Many of the interviewees expressed views about the concept of a patient-centred approach to planning and organising the health services of the future. The move to more primary care-based services was seen as central. But a policymaker expressed the hope that, in this move, 'that nurses don't lose [sight of the fact that] the patient is at the centre and that they have the responsibility for everything that surrounds the patient'.

The role of the nurse as an advocate for the patient occurs frequently throughout the research and will be covered in later chapters. It is an important dimension of a move towards increased awareness of the need for a patient-centred approach to the development of high-quality services:

> Service manager: Not alone do nurses have the missing element to bring to that, but they can maybe bring a little bit more patient-orientation to it and that's not in any way to insult the other professions that are involved.

The Cultural Challenge

All categories of interviewees were quite clear about the importance of a cultural change in the health services of the future (see Table 13) – and recognised that this would take time. The changes in culture required within the health services of the future are driven by the demands of the changes that have been examined throughout this chapter and the issue of culture is one that arises throughout this research and will recur in later chapters when we look at the themes of role change, education and skills.

Table 13: Research Issues: Cultural Challenge

Theme	Frequency of mention
The future health services will present a significant cultural challenge	24
The requirement for increased interdisciplinarity in service delivery requires the development of a new culture	66
The need for increased teamworking requires the creation and development of a new culture	62
The relationship between the professions is an important part of the cultural change need for future health services	19
The demands of future health service delivery will require the breaking down of the silos in which professions have traditionally operated	29

The biggest change in culture that is required is in the area of teamworking and interdisciplinary working relationships between professionals. One service manager noted that medical errors quite frequently occur at the interface between the disciplines (professional, management, administrative and clerical) and that, therefore, the need for teams is driven by the need to reduce the potential for this kind of error to occur:

> Service manager: We are terribly hierarchical, very focused on our individual disciplines and all the literature shows that major medical errors (and we have a lot of them) don't occur necessarily within the disciplines but at the interface between the disciplines, whether it be doctors and nurses or the anaesthetists and surgeons or managers and professionals. It's because they don't talk to each other and because professionals particularly, and it's true for doctors, aren't trained to the notion of teamworking and communication and that's where most of the problems arise.

In considering the composition of multidisciplinary teams, the interviewees also made the point that the medical professionals do not always necessarily lead teams. There is a perception generally that the medics see themselves as natural team leaders and that may not be so in the future:

> Educator: I think the challenges are to really get teams working well, to set up things like care pathways where everybody has big responsibilities and the teams work well. It also sets the challenges for the medics because the leader of the team does not necessarily have to be a medic and that is something that we have to really work on.

Interviewees also spoke about the importance of inculcating an interdisciplinary instinct as part of the normal way of doing business. One policymaker referred to making the 'interdisciplinary instinct part of the basic toolkit of any healing professional'.

Working as part of an interdisciplinary team and improving the relationships between the professionals and other disciplines is an essential ingredient in improving the patient's journey, the quality of care. Interviewees who referred to the concept of 'the patient's journey' also believed, in the words of an NMPDU director, that where 'multidisciplinary teamworking worked really well, it did improve the patient's journey'.

Within the services, nurses are generally seen as being well disposed to interdisciplinary teamworking. There is also ample evidence from this research that clinicians are positively disposed to working in teams, with one medical consultant describing multidisciplinary working as 'core', and identifying one of the problems of working in teams where, to quote a medical consultant, 'doctors are more assertive, nurses are more assertive, physiotherapists, occupational therapists are more assertive:

everybody is more assertive and more certain that their view is right'. The interviewee believed that this makes working in teams more challenging.

The creation of the HSE and the potential that it presents for a more integrated approach across the whole health care system is something that was seen as potentially contributing greatly towards the development of this culture of cross-discipline teamworking. Some interviewees felt that interdisciplinary teamworking would significantly influence the way in which the development and delivery of services are organised. For example:

> Regulator: The antiquated nature of our outpatient systems means that 80 per cent of those attending outpatients are still repeat visitors who largely have limited or no interventions carried out and are in the system simply because they are in the system. It seems to me that, if we were to radically reduce the recurrent stable patient from those systems, and if we were to ensure that outpatients were to be used for specialist advice on difficult problems or new presentations and if were to have systems in place to control the patients with diabetes, hypertension, epilepsy, asthma, all of the other problems that cause our chronic disease problems at the moment, if those patients were better managed by an interdisciplinary approach, we would have better organisation all around and I think nursing has a profound role to play in all of that.

Interdisciplinary working is also an essential ingredient of the hospital accreditation process that has become so valued in recent years. One service manager remarked: 'The concept of accreditation is an interdisciplinary approach to the evaluation'. Accreditation, therefore, looks at the interaction of all the disciplines in a hospital setting, including clinical and non-clinical staff.

From all categories a common message emerged. One interviewee summed it up as follows:

> Service manager: We are moving towards a multidisciplinary method of service delivery with more of an emphasis on collaborative working, more of an awareness of what other professions can do, less emphasis on demarcation and more of a move towards common decision-making as well.

Conclusions

It is possible to identify a number of key conclusions of what the health services of the future in Ireland will be like based on the comments of interviewees and on the research outlined in the earlier chapters of this book. Many of these conclusions mirror the conclusions already identified in Chapters 3 and 4. They can be summarised in the following points:

- The health services of the future will be delivered to a population that will be wealthier, with higher expectations about what they can expect from public services. This affluence will generate a culture where patients and clients expect services to be delivered without the need to wait and to a high standard of quality and personal service.
- Consumers of health services will place a large emphasis on value for money from the services. They will be more informed about what constitutes 'good service' and will demand a higher quality of service. This will change radically the relationship between the consumer and the service provider and between the consumer and clinical professionals. The leaders of the services of the future will need to give consideration to the changes in expectations of consumers in the development of service infrastructure. 'More of the same' will not be acceptable.
- Ireland's population will continue to grow at a fast rate and the birth rate will continue to increase. This means that there will be a higher demand for health services that are adapted to the profile of the population.
- Health service consumers are concerned about how older people will be treated within the health services of the future. This is further exacerbated by changes in the structure of the family and the disappearance of traditional support structures. This has significant implications for the health services and the nature of support that can be provided to carers and to people in their own homes.
- The population of the future will be working more, with a higher level of female participation in the workforce. This will lead to further fragmentation in the nature of family relationships and the existing support structures.
- Increased wealth will bring with it an increase in lifestyle diseases such as obesity, diabetes, and alcohol- and drug-related illnesses.
- The population of Ireland will continue to become more ethnically and culturally diverse. This has implications for

the delivery of services and in particular the need for sensitivity to cultural differences and communication issues. It also raises questions for recruitment practices within the services and the need for increased training for professionals and administrators in dealing with a more diverse population and consumer base.

- The health services of the future will be delivered by a single, integrated accountable entity. It will lead to a greater degree of accountability within the system. The creation of the HSE should lead to a greater equality of access to services and to the development of higher standards in the delivery of services. The HSE is likely to face pressure for increased integration of services and administrative structures and, in particular, to revise the division between the two pillars: PCCC and NHO. The structures as they are currently configured are more suitable for bureaucratic control and distribution of funding resources than for service delivery management. They are also not conducive to the clinical management of services. (As already noted, in July 2008 the HSE announced, as part of plans to speed up service integration, that the NHO and PCCC will come under the leadership of a single national director of integrated service delivery.)
- In order to make progress in the integration of services, there is a need to review the involvement of clinical leaders at all levels of the health service delivery structures. This is required not only to assist in the integration of services, but also to ensure that clinical safety is an integral part of the decision-making process within the system. This may require the creation of posts at national and regional level for clinical coordination, involving hospitals and primary care teams. A clustering system may be appropriate with a view to bringing together primary care and hospital structures within regional and local geographic areas. (See page 61, HSE appointment of national director of clinical care and quality.)
- This entails major changes for the role of the Department of Health and Children and will drive cultural changes in areas such as political accountability. It will require the development of new relationships with the HSE, inspired by the principles of performance management, public safety and value for money. As is the case for the HSE, clinical safety

will need to become an integral part of the procedures and processes involved in policy formulation and performance monitoring.

- The creation of the HSE should lead to greater equality of access to services and to the development of higher standards in the delivery of services.
- The health services of the future will see acute hospitals focus entirely on major acute interventions. Service delivery will shift to the primary care setting in the community, with an increase in initiatives such as the hospital in the home (HITH) and community intervention teams (CIT).
- The shift of emphasis towards primary care settings has implications for health care professionals. They will follow the patient into the community and most of them will be working in community bases rather than acute hospital settings. This has also implications for the education and training of professionals.
- Patients and consumers of health care services can expect to receive more services within their own homes and within their own communities, delivered by professionals who are based in the community. Many services will be nurse-/midwife-led. There will be a system of primary care-based interdisciplinary and multidisciplinary teams, including and sometimes led by the GP.
- Nurses and midwives within the community will be expected to link together better and to link with other professionals as part of multidisciplinary primary care teams.
- There will be an increase in the number and nature of 'networked' hospitals, involving close links between various hospitals and academic institutions.
- There will be an increase in the availability of diagnostic and assessment services that do not require admission to hospitals. Length of stay in hospital will be shorter and there will be more protocol-based early discharge arrangements in place. Professionals will follow up with the patient in the community.
- There will be an increase in the provision of private health services. Consumers will be offered and will avail of greater choice.
- The health services of the future will be delivered with a very high emphasis on personal and professional accountability

within the system. This has implications for managers and clinical professionals within the system, who will expect to be accountable for their area of service delivery and be called to account for the value for money of their services.

- Standards in both private and public health care provision will be driven by HIQA and the respective regulatory bodies of the different professions. This will mean a major increase in the quantity and intensity of audit within the system, with consequences for the way professionals account for their work.
- Political pressure will increase for evidence of value for money in the provision of public finances for health services.
- The health services of the future will be delivered in an environment where clients/consumers/patients are more empowered. They will be in possession of more information, of a higher quality and will expect to be treated as equals in discussing the services they require. This has implications for the relationships between patient or consumer and health care professionals and administrators. It also has implications for the quality of services that will be expected.
- The services of the future will be driven by a greater and more widespread use of technology, in particular information and communications technology. This will lead to an increase in the level of technology-driven services, the availability of e-health options and the networking of professionals and systems across institutional boundaries. It will underpin the increased emphasis on community-based services and remote consultation.
- Nursing and midwifery will have an important role in continuing to act as an advocate for the patient in what will become a patient-centred health service, with emphasis on integrated care pathways and the patient's journey.
- The development of the health services of the future will require a transformation of the culture of the nursing and midwifery professions. In particular, it will demand a multidisciplinary method of service delivery, a greater emphasis on collaborative working, a greater awareness of what other professions can do, less emphasis on demarcation and a move towards common decision-making.

CHAPTER 9

Research Results: The Changing Role of Nursing and Midwifery

The second part of the research moved the focus from an assessment of the future of the Irish health services to the more specific topic of whether, and in what ways, the professions of nursing and midwifery are going to change over the next ten years. Interviewees responded to five pertinent questions:

- Do you think the role of nurses and midwives will change significantly over the next ten years?
- In what way do you think the new role will differ from the current role?
- Do you think general managers and nurse/midwife managers understand the way in which the role of nurses and midwives will change?
- In what way will the relationships between the various professions and grades involved in the delivery of the health services change in the future?
- What are your opinions of the current level of preparedness of nurses and midwives for the challenges ahead?

The changing role for nurses and midwives was discussed under six broad themes:

1. Clinical career pathways
2. Adaptation to role change
3. Leadership
4. Nurse-/midwife-led services
5. Interdisciplinary teams
6. Relationship between primary and acute care services.

Clinical Career Pathways

The most frequent themes regarding clinical career pathways are summarised in Table 14. There was strong agreement among all

Table 14: Research Issues: Clinical Career Pathways

Theme	Frequency of mention
There is a need for more specialist nurses in future health services	75
Increased specialisation in nursing has some inherent disadvantages	18
ANPs and AMPs are an important dimension of specialisation and role change for nurses and midwives	46
Specialist nurses will need to develop new relationships with medical consultants	2
The existence of more specialist nurses and midwives will require an examination of the changes in the relationships with non-consultant hospital doctors	13
It is important to provide staff nurses and staff midwives with access to a meaningful clinical career pathway	9

interviewees that increased specialisation is both necessary and good for nursing. It was also seen as following best international practice.

Service managers commented that new medical consultants frequently expect to be allocated a CNS or ANP. In some instances, they even express a preference for specialist nurses over junior doctors. Where ANPs had not yet been introduced, new incoming medical consultants, particularly those who had worked abroad, often created the demand:

> Service manager: I have noticed in recent years that if new medical consultants come, the first thing they look for is a CNS. I have noticed this when medical consultants have their shopping list and that is a clear indication to me that CNSs play an absolutely vital role in service provision. This will become even more important going forward with the European Working Time Directive.

Interviewees commented on how the implementation of the EWTD would impact on the clinical career pathway for nurses and midwives and the opportunities that this might mean for the development of their role.

Medical consultants saw the advantages of more specialists and the role they could fulfil in relation to the implementation of the working time directive. In addition to the benefits of having nurse specialists, one medical consultant commented:

> Nurse specialists are now taking over roles that, to a degree, were fulfilled by doctors before, particularly junior doctors. But now nurses can

> run clinics and there are actually huge advantages to it because you have continuity, you can work within an agreed pathway of protocols.

The same was true in midwifery, where medical consultants spoke about the benefits of having clinical midwifery specialists.

Medical consultants see the ANP as a welcome expansion of the role of the nurse, who does not replace the role of the medical practitioner but better enables it, and has become increasingly indispensable in certain areas of service provision.

> Medical consultant: We couldn't survive without ANPs. We have advanced nurse practitioners here or CNSs and they are all the time involved with the patients, explaining the use of the drug, the use of the syringe, how to give it, if there are any problems to contact them, and all of that. So it enables a service that would not otherwise be as effective.

Clearly, specialist and advanced practice nurses are seen as enabling services to be provided that would otherwise not be provided and add significantly to the overall effectiveness of the clinical team, to the decision-making process and to the delivery of services.

Interviewees with a nursing background were generally very favourably disposed towards the idea of increased specialisation within the professions and were in favour of the role of CNSs and ANPs. They also felt that, as the specialist roles developed into other areas and, in particular, once audits of their work were undertaken and disseminated, the real benefits of this approach would become apparent.

The directors of the NMPDUs also mentioned the potential for nurse specialists to provide support to nurses in more generalist roles. There was a need for balance, and the role of the generalist nurse in the clinical area was seen as very important. A service manager made this comment:

> Specialisation is important. I accept that and it goes without saying, but there is a need for someone who, as a generalist, knows who to call or when to call.

The directors of nursing and midwifery also emphasised the great contribution nurse specialists were making to the overall quality of clinical services and would welcome their wider involvement outside their specialist clinics and in the general areas to lead nursing care. Said one:

> I think we will see increased specialisation. We have already seen the advantages of having specialist nurses. They bring a huge change in the quality of care that is delivered to patients, and the specialist knowledge that is brought to the wards has changed so much as a result of having specialist nurses on the ground. I would really like to see them become more involved in clinical practice with the generalist nurse, as opposed to being isolated in their own clinic and their own specialty area, and that we try and bring them out there to enhance care more because they are really good.

The directors of nursing and midwifery related this to the idea put forward by Patricia Benner in *Novice to Expert*,[243] where the specialist nurses play the role of experts in helping novices along the pathway and use their judgment to address the many critical issues nurses and midwives face on a daily basis within the clinical area. Benner also introduced the idea of 'clinical wisdom' and 'clinical judgement' as part of the characteristics of an expert nurse:

> Director of nursing and midwifery: I suppose the *Novice to Expert* model is a very good one; that they have the skills, depending on what level they are at. I think one of the mistakes we make is that we are not looking at the years of qualification that nurses have. But we do have novices out there and there is a reluctance on the more experienced nurses to develop those novices and bring them along and I think we have to focus on that much more in the future.

However, most interviewees with a nursing background saw the move towards specialisation as evidence of nurses taking a greater leadership role in the clinical area:

> Educator: In CNS and ANP development, I see many more nurses taking on responsibility and contributing within the service areas and really looking at taking on leadership roles.

The move towards increased specialisation within nursing raises the important question of measurement of impact and effectiveness:

> Service manager: Once people are specialists they need constantly to be monitored. That is important because people are going to be judged by outcomes and how is all this achieving a better service for the public? How is it contributing to greater accessibility for patients? And that, really, will be the final arbiter in deciding whether or not nurses can meet the challenges and whether or not any changes that have been proposed have been effective.

Adaptation to Role Change

Interviewees discussed adaptation to role change in the health services under eight headings (see Table 15). Interviewees saw adaptation to change as a positive outcome. A number said that it would be important to provide nurses and midwives with career guidance.

Table 15: Research Issues: Adaptation to Role Change

Theme	Frequency of mention
Nurses and midwives need to be proactive in adapting to role changes	24
The clinical career pathway is an important element of adapting to change in role changes for nurses and midwives	21
There is a need for nurses and midwives to become involved in prescribing as part of the future role change for nurses and midwives	51
Are nurses and midwives prepared for the changes ahead?	74
Do nurse managers have a good understanding of the way the role of nurses and midwives will change?	48
Do general managers have a good understanding of the way in which the role of nurses and midwives will change?	47
There is a problem of resistance to change within nursing and midwifery, particularly in relation to changes of role	21
There is a problem of resistance to change from within the trade unions that represent nursing and midwifery	37

As with their comments on clinical career pathways, interviewees saw adaptation to change as a positive outcome for nursing resulting from the work of the Commission on Nursing. However, a number said that it would be important to provide nurses and midwives with some career guidance, counselling or support services in order to encourage them to reflect on the career pathway that would suit them best. This would, from an economic perspective, ensure better value for money from the investment in their training and development, trying to ensure that they did not spend a long time in a career path that did not suit them.

Career guidance would also ensure that nurses who are particularly suited to management or clinical career pathways, or who might be better involved in education, professional development or research, would have an opportunity to find this out sooner rather than later in their careers and be facilitated to take the better path. This raised the possibility of pathways other than clinical career pathways. Mention was made of opportunities in management, education, research and professional development. In order to ensure that nursing and midwifery adapt to change in a proactive manner, career advice and support on these issues was seen by participants as important, especially early in their career.

Interviewees said that nurses and midwives should take advantage of opportunities under the emerging strategies for the development of primary care services and the extension of the roles of nurses and midwives to proactively adapt and lead the change in these areas.

Comments on nurse and midwife prescribing were made in the context of the national review that was being conducted at the time on the involvement of nurses and midwives in the prescribing of medicines (see page 32). As a result, there was a high degree of awareness within the health services of this issue and it is not surprising that most interviewees referred directly to it.

There was unanimous agreement that the involvement of nurses and midwives in prescribing was both desirable and inevitable. At a policy level, this was already happening in other areas of the health services, and it made no sense not to do something similar in nursing and midwifery. One policymaker commented:

> Progress has already been made on the medical technicians where a statutory instrument is being prepared to allow certain drugs to be given in emergency situations.

Many of the interviewees believed that there was a need for 'proper' training and education to give the required degree of confidence that a particular person was a competent practitioner to prescribe. They also considered that prescribing should not be confined to a limited number of medications (the list method):

> Service manager: People talk about minor things like Panadol and whatever, but I see it as a lot more; in a lot of cases, there is no reason why psychiatric nurses cannot prescribe appropriate medication. In many instances, they would have a lot more experience with psychiatric patients out of hours than some of the junior doctors; the same in paediatrics; the same in ICU.

Similarly, medical consultants in areas such as midwifery and care of the elderly supported the idea of nurses and midwives having a wide role in prescribing, provided they had the appropriate education, training and certification.

Interviewees also considered the pros and cons of limiting prescribing to CNSs and ANPs. The present research reflected the lack of consensus on this issue identified in the international literature. Thus, for example, one NMPDU director felt that 'you are looking at your ANP level being involved in the prescribing process'; and another, a medical consultant, saw it as 'a perfectly logical extension of a specialist role'. On the other hand, one of the trade union representative interviewees expressed the hope that the development of these skills and competencies would not be confined to an elite group of nurses and that it would be done in a way that empowered the staff nurse. Other participants agreed. The involvement of nurses and midwives in prescribing was seen as a logical extension of the other changes in the delivery of services and the role that they would be expected to play within it. A service manager summed up the overall view succinctly: 'I don't think nursing will move very far unless nurses move into areas of prescribing and they are central to the new ways of working'. Some interviewees from the policy, service managers and medical consultants' groups went further, indicating their support for the involvement of nurses and midwives in ordering radiology and laboratory services.

Interviewees were split approximately 60:40 on the statement that nurses and midwives were prepared for change. But, in expanding on the topic, a slightly less clear-cut picture emerged. As another service manager put it, 'the vast majority are sheep following the shepherd and that is the normal frequency distribution; most of them in the centre; there are a few out there'.

While the interviewees used expressions like 'patchy', and 'somewhat', and 'don't know for sure', the overall impression from each of the interview groups was positive. Thus, for example, one service manager said:

> Nursing has probably been the area where people have become most aware of the need for change and it is still a long way behind what we require. But I think nurses are a long way ahead of other therapists in terms of understanding that their role is going to change. I think that

> the whole CNS and advanced practitioner model is now very well understood.

Many mentioned the impact of the work of the Commission on Nursing and the role of the National Council in implementing the clinical career pathways, the value and impact of the introduction of the degree programme in education, and the likelihood that changes in education would further enhance the image of nurses and midwives.

Similarly, the point was made that those who have participated in continuing professional development activities, which are seen generally as beginning to have an impact, are much more aware and have a greater understanding of the role changes that are happening. The value of postgraduate training was also mentioned as contributing to this awareness, particularly the fact that more nurse managers have masters' degrees in such areas as nursing, midwifery or health care management or business administration, and other similarly regarded qualifications.

Medical consultants shared the same realism about preparedness. However, they also spoke about a cohort of nurses and midwives who, to quote one, 'are not heavily into the academic side of nursing and they are... disappointed. They feel marginalised'.

Nurse interviewees tended to agree and voiced concerns about the extent of the awareness within the professions, and about how big the cohorts were that were prepared for change. They also questioned the extent to which nurses and midwives were engaged in continuing professional development activities or postgraduate education. As one director of NMPDU said:

> It is worrying sometimes because we are in the middle of the biggest change ever in the State.

Those involved in education were, perhaps, closer to the cohort that is more likely to be prepared. They, too, sounded a note of caution:

> Educator: We are partially there but, at the same time, I think that nurses are a funny group because sometimes we are so rigid and so reactionary and yet look at what we have coped with over the last twenty or thirty years.

What emerges is a realistic picture of a large group of professionals working in a system that is undergoing extensive, far-reaching and protracted transition. Awareness levels are what one would expect and are contingent on factors such as the degree of involvement in education, professional development and the roles in which they are engaged.

Many interviewees spoke about initiatives that were in place to inform the professions about emerging changes:

> Director of NMPDU: We meet up with the directors three or four times a year and they are fully briefed and I know our own practice development people are working very closely with the assistant directors, divisional nurse managers and CNM2s.

The directors of the NMPDUs also spoke about the work they do with the general managers, including, for example, encouraging them to participate in briefing sessions and attend the national conference of the National Council, which is seen as an important dimension of building understanding and buy-in. They accepted that the level of understanding at general management level was a challenge:

> NMPDU director: For general managers, whether or not they understand will depend largely upon us as nurse leaders in how we influence them.

Similarly, educators within nursing spoke of the opportunity for leadership within the professions (administrative, managerial, professional and education) to develop understanding within nursing and within general management. Nevertheless, directors of NMPDUs commented that there was still a lack of understanding about how the relationship between nurse management and general management needed to change. There was a lack of clarity about the sharing of responsibility and the complementary nature of their roles. This was seen as a fault on both sides and evidence of confusion within nursing itself about its overall role in management.

One NMPDU director spoke about an experience of interviewing a very competent and highly skilled nurse, with experience in a system where she had budgetary control and was used to making decisions as a key player within a directorate system. The director asked the general manager who was interviewing: 'Are you ready for her? If you don't embrace what she has, she will be gone'.

Some medical consultants who have already developed good working relations with their general management and nursing and midwifery colleagues spoke enthusiastically about the understanding that existed regarding the changes that needed to take place. Others, however, mentioned their frustration at the lack of understanding of change that is needed at both general management and nursing management levels.

Finally, from the service manager group came an opinion that it was only when one saw something working that real understanding occurred and so the emphasis had to be on getting things moving and not waiting for everybody to understand.

Resistance to change as an issue largely emerged spontaneously from unsolicited comments made by interviewees from within the professions of nursing and midwifery and as a result of the involvement of trade unions. A number of interviewees reflected on the role of the trade unions at the time of the publication of the *Report of the Commission on Nursing* in 1998. In 1999, the Government had not implemented the Commission's recommendations and nurses voted for strike action. The strike lasted from 19 October to 27 October 1999. At the time, many nurses expressed dissatisfaction with the way the strike had been handled, including the initiation, management and outcome of the strike; they felt that a different approach could have achieved more. Some interviewees in this research argued that the strike emphasised the power of the unions and resulted in the role of the director of nursing and midwifery being marginalised.

A number spoke about the pressure from trade unions on senior nurse and midwife managers. As a result, many directors of nursing and assistant directors of nursing had resisted the introduction of change because of the fear of falling foul of the unions. Interviewees also believed that the trade unions had too much influence on the wider nursing and midwifery professions and were not a beneficial influence; they held the professions back and resisted change. One service manager referred to 'being dictated to by a lot of males, who are looking at their own [trade union] careers rather than the totality of the profession'.

Overwhelmingly, the picture was of professions that had become too preoccupied with industrial relations agendas, were dominated by trade unions, were fearful of change and were too ready to row back on progress and change that had already been made. These views were expressed by all categories of interviewees, and should be balanced by the more positive views expressed by interviewees when talking about nursing and midwifery's general ability to adapt to change.

The reality of continued industrial disputes and complaints had created bitterness in some quarters. For example, a service manager commented:

> The changes I had hoped to see arising from the Commission are not obvious and I don't see signs that they are going to happen. That is a perception from a distance but it would also be a perception that I hear talked about.

And a policymaker observed:

> So 1998 was the Commission on Nursing and 1998/99 was the industrial relations problem. Nothing moved. Effectively, things started rolling towards the end of 1999/2000. The profession itself is still coming to terms with that. Maybe at some stage we need to step back and have a look critically at where we are going: have we done it right? Are there changes needed?

In the focus groups, the directors of nursing and midwifery lamented the slow pace of implementation and the negative effect that the industrial relations issues had had on this. However, most believed that the Commission on Nursing had lifted nursing and midwifery in Ireland onto a new level. Nurses and midwives were also aware that not enough has changed in the style of management within nursing:

> Director of NMPDU: I'd like to say that the impact of the Commission on Nursing has been huge but the 'command and control' style of management still exists in some areas, particularly mental health nursing and community nursing.

The reference to 'command and control' style of nursing raises memories of the harsh criticisms that were made of nurse management in the *Interim Report of the Commission on Nursing*.[244] At the time, nurse management was characterised as being predominantly old-style, with a lot of bullying in evidence within the services. According to the *Interim Report* (3.1): 'many nurses complained of bullying in the workplace.... It appeared that bullying may be taking place at a variety of levels within nursing. Complaints were made of students being bullied by nurses, nurses being bullied by other nurses and professionals, nurses being bullied by nurse management and nurse management being bullied by general management'. The vision of management for nursing provided in the *Report of the Commission on Nursing* was intended to move beyond that. When commenting on issues in senior nurse management, the report said: 'it was suggested that senior nursing and midwifery management operated on the basis of command and control rather than consultation and the delegation of responsibility'.

Some service managers, in particular, expressed considerable frustration with the focus on industrial relations issues within the professions. For example:

> Service manager: Nursing is much too industrial relations-focused and the profession is hampered by that obsession with industrial relations.

The same interviewee also spoke about the lack of confidence within the system in nursing's ability to tackle these issues. Whenever an industrial relations issue arose, the first things that suffered were the professional development advances that had already been achieved. They were used as tools in the industrial relations negotiation process. Nurses stopped doing what their professional development advances had introduced. This, the interviewee said, frequently also led to legalistic interpretation of guidelines, which, in some cases, made it impossible to deal with practical issues on the ground for the benefit of patients.

Service managers commented on the slow pace of professional development. For example:

> Service manager: The development and evolution of nursing as a profession will not be addressed by the industrial relations arm of the profession... they have a vested interest in blocking the candid development that would allow nursing as a profession to be of the highly skilled kind.

The issue comes back to leadership in nursing and the lack of it. Interviewees commented on the leadership on the industrial relations side of nursing and regretted that the same energy and leadership frequently was not evident in the development of the scope and practice of the professions. The trade unions had dominated the professional development debate in the past and used it for industrial relations purposes rather than for the benefit of the professions as professions. This was because the leadership was not available within nursing and midwifery; the leadership competencies were not there. There was a recognition that this had changed with the arrival of the National Council:

> Service manager: In the absence of a body like the National Council in the past, the unions, or interests like trade unions, saw an opportunity.

Nurses also recognised that there was a strong union influence at local level that was impeding change and progress. One director of NMPDU said: 'we do have a strong culture of militancy and unions within the service... that needs to be addressed'.

A number of service managers spoke about the difficulty of getting nurses to cooperate during a strike to cover genuine emergency cases. According to one:

> It came home to me in the last negotiation I had around the A&E strike, when I almost had to beg to get emergency cover for the patients.

Another mentioned the example of introducing health care assistants and talked of nurses 'holding onto their territory' and 'protecting old boundaries'.

Service managers also expressed frustration at the inability of nurse management to identify with management in industrial relations disputes. The interviewees said that nursing unions constantly criticised 'the management' for all of the problems that they saw, but did not take account of the fact that nurses and midwives formed a large cohort of 'the management'. Nursing management, in turn, was cowed by the power of the unions and fearful of stepping up to the line to tackle industrial relations issues from a management perspective.

> Service manager: It is as though it is not their responsibility; they don't see their managerial role as having any particular relevance, or it is as though they are playing down their managerial role.

Some linked the pressure that is on nurse managers in this area with the difficulty that is experienced in attracting applicants for some senior nursing management posts. A service manager noted, 'people are not going into management roles or taking on other roles because of the sheer pressure and demand that comes on them'.

Nurses were deterred from applying for nursing management posts and nurse managers were reluctant to take on the management role because of the culture that exists beneath them and that rises up against them. Service managers spoke about the need for this culture to change but expressed frustration at the ability to change, with some saying that they did not detect an ability to change it within the professions. Those who did speak about how to change said that it should be done through education and motivational feedback.

Policymakers referred to 'the voice of nursing' in public and said that this 'voice' had become a 'constant whine' about monetary and status issues. They saw a dearth of leadership in nursing management, and one commented that:

> Nurse management at the moment is poorly organised. The best organised element of nursing at the moment is the INO [Irish Nurses Organisation], SIPTU [Services, Industrial, Professional and Technical Union] and the PNA [Psychiatric Nurses Association]... but from my desk I would see that they have adopted a very negative role.

Medical consultants spoke about their frustration at introducing change and being suspected of 'trying to off-load work'. They also commented that nursing was frequently 'driven by union concerns' and that this was not helping the professions.

Nursing and midwifery will face increased demands to adapt to change as a result of the recommendations made on the resolution of the industrial dispute that took place in 2007. The dispute was principally about the reduction of the working week for nurses and midwives from the current thirty-nine hours per week to thirty-five hours per week. The dispute concluded with a recommendation that a phased approach would be taken to the reduction in working hours. Phase 1 entailed the reduction in hours to 37.5 by 1 June 2008. Phase 2 involved the setting up of a Commission to examine the feasibility of reducing the working week to thirty-five hours. Both Phase 1 and Phase 2 will entail changes in roles and working practices for nurses and midwives.

Emerging Leadership

The need for leadership within nursing was, after accountability, the second most frequently mentioned topic throughout the whole of this research. It is perhaps even more interesting given that interviewees raised it spontaneously. On this subject, interviewees discussed four broad issues, as summarised in Table 16.

Table 16: Research Issues: Emerging Leadership

Theme	Frequency of mention
There is a great need for leaders to emerge from within nursing and midwifery	125
Empowerment is an important dimension in role change	20
Nurses need to learn to be more assertive in their relationships with medical consultants and others within the services	51
There are a number of issues arising in relation to the involvement of nurses and midwives in management, including the general management of services and the management of nursing and midwifery	52

Both policymaker and service manager interviewees expressed the opinion that nursing management had not stepped up to the mark in the way that it had been hoped they would after the *Report of the Commission on Nursing*. Nurse managers themselves believed they were let down by the outcome of the recommendations of the Commission, ending up more isolated in their role as managers and still not integrated into the key decision-making mechanisms.

From the service point of view, nurses were seen as not being assertive enough:

> Policymaker: Nurse managers need to be pushing their way in management and putting their hand up and saying 'look we have experience of the business that nobody else can match'. I think that, to a large extent, nurses aren't as assertive in those areas of management as they should be and as befits their experience.

There seemed still to be confusion about the role of the director of nursing. Is it strategic? What about the operational side? What is the role of the assistant director of nursing (ADON) and CNM3? There was a lack of understanding and of support for the important roles of the ADON and CNM3 in particular. As a result, according to one service manager, there was confusion about applying for such posts and a lack of support for those who hold them and those who aspire to them.

Interviewees frequently made reference to the management structure for nursing and midwifery that has been in place since the Commission on Nursing, with many voicing concerns about the lack of clarity of the roles and the increasing complexity of management structures.

Some interviewees spoke of the role of educators in influencing thinking within nursing about the meaning and implications of leadership, accountability and responsibility. One service manager thought that educators should be influencing the career development of students as they came into the system, but they should also be working with more senior personnel in preparing them for their roles as innovative accountable leaders.

An important function of nurse leaders, said another service manager, was acting as advocates for nursing staff. In the absence of good leadership from nurse management, nurses and midwives were turning to their staff associations and unions for leadership and advocacy on their behalf.

Service managers defined the lack of leadership in nursing as a lack of advocacy for nursing, making strong statements about how nursing should position itself within the services, such as:

> I do not see leaders in the nursing profession in the way that I do in the medical profession, for example. I think there is an issue there. I don't know what the reason for that is. It seems to me that nursing is quite passive in terms of setting the vision for nursing for the future, that nursing leadership is not setting out the vision for nursing into the future. Nursing leadership in this country should be taking that debate forward in the interests of the profession.

This service manager hoped that nursing and midwifery would produce leaders who would analyse the environment, understand the changes and make strong statements about how nursing and midwifery should be positioned within it, in cooperation with – but not deferring to – the medical profession, and not waiting for the leadership to come from the unions. The only leadership that was prominent in nursing and midwifery was frequently industrial relations-orientated, leaving a major gap in the development of the professions. This accorded with the views already noted about resistance to change.

This interviewee went on to suggest that the kind of leadership that was needed must emerge from within nursing itself and should be coordinated between nursing management, nursing academics and other nurse leaders, and linked to other functions. This kind of integrated planning for leadership was not happening at present:

> I think it needs fundamentally to begin with nurses and that leadership of nursing needs to be given by nurses. I have no doubt at all about that and there is a need for close linkages between the academic units and the senior management units and collaboration at the academic units between the nursing schools and medical schools and between the management side.

Directors of nursing and midwifery agreed. They spoke about the need for nursing management to change and become more strategic and that if this change did not happen they would be left in 'little pockets':

> Nursing will not develop unless we lead the change and I think it will remain stagnant unless we are looking at very innovative ways of trying to create the seamless service that we feel is going to be missing in the new structures. We have to see how we can develop specialisation on maybe a shared basis between acute and community services so that we are looking at ANPs going out maybe, for example, looking at the elderly. This would mean that they are not hospital-based nor community-based but are a shared responsibility. They would be looking at a specialist service throughout at regional level, as opposed to just focused in a hospital, and maybe they could look at needs on a population basis, as opposed to just on the actual acute or community service basis. Unless we are looking at that strategically, and in a much broader basis than what we are doing currently, we will be just left in the little pockets we are in.

When meetings were organised by one part of the nursing and midwifery professions, very often it was done without adequately informing or involving the other. According to one educator:

> I find it amazing that, for example, the directors of the NMPDUs would have meetings with the directors of nursing and not automatically include the higher education institutions. Part of the reason for that is that [nurses working] in universities [are] still seen as purveyors of courses rather than people who understand anything about the health service or who can feed into it in terms of research or ideas or in a think-tank kind of set-up.

There is an idea in this comment of a 'think-tank for nursing', involving all of the key stakeholders and providing the opportunity for inputs from the various nursing areas (clinical, management, education, professional development and regulation) into the formulation of a vision for nursing – taking the lead in providing the leadership that is being called for. This is required despite the fact that frequently there is a sense that people feel 'swamped'. In educational circles, for example, all effort in recent years has been directed towards setting up the degree programmes and postgraduate programmes recommended by the Commission on Nursing.

This raises the question about the relationships between the different elements involved in nursing throughout the service. Relationships are not always easy and, in the case of the relationships between the directors of nursing and the NMPDUs, there is work to be done in clarifying the ways in which they work together:

> Service manager: The relationship between the NMPDUs and the directors of nursing is a difficult one and I think that if we can manage to resolve that we can help to empower them a little bit more.

It also raises questions about the relationships between the different groups of nurse managers, between the directors of nursing in Band 1 hospitals through to Band 5 hospitals, and between the various levels of nurse management, i.e. between directors of nursing and other nursing management grades. There is evidence to suggest that divisions exist between the bands and the grades that are not serving the purposes of the professions well.

Interviewees spoke about elitism and a hierarchy within nursing, wherein directors of Band 1 hospitals saw themselves as being at the top of a notional pyramid and would occasionally involve directors of nursing from Band 2 hospitals, but would never have anything to do with directors of nursing from Bands 3, 4 and 5. Similarly, directors of nursing and their associations would not engage directly with the associations of other nurse managers – the Irish Association of Directors of Nursing and Midwifery (IADNAM) and ENTRUST, the association of nurse managers at CNM1, CNM2, CNM3 and assistant director levels.

> Policymaker: There is no unifying structure, even where they could come together as a federation of nurse managers and say, 'look, we as nurse managers play a huge role in keeping this show on the road, we are not always listened to, we don't get our hands on lots of the budgets and we should draw up an agenda to make sure that we are in there at the table'.

This interviewee suggested that there was a need for a more united front and more strategic coordination from nursing management that was different from the industrial relations-based negotiations that take place. This would require the breaking down of silos within the professions.

Some of the service managers said that the Commission on Nursing did not tackle the question of integrating nursing management into the wider decision-making structures within the services, leaving it isolated. One way to do this would be a more concerted, coordinated approach to articulating the 'nursing voice' in a manner that would lift it beyond just the nursing dimension and takes account of the wider issues within the services.

The strategic voice of nursing was not being heard across a multidisciplinary range of areas in the way that the Commission on Nursing envisaged that it would be. One service manager observed:

> I don't see a strategic sense of influence within the Department. I see an awful lot of excellent work done but I don't see a very strong policy influence in terms of the multidisciplinary health service as opposed to the nursing one. Nurses have not played their part, as I think it was envisaged that they would almost be part of the broader influencing of a strategic approach to the health services from a multidisciplinary point of view. Now maybe they were not allowed to do it or maybe there was not an acceptance by virtue of where it came from in terms of the idea being put into place. I am not sure that they are at the table other than at the industrial relations area of nursing.

This reflects a view among interviewees that the strategic role of the policy unit within the Department of Health and Children was not being felt within the professions or within the health services generally. The role of the chief nurse within the Department needed, according to a number of interviewees, to be re-defined, particularly in light of the changes that had taken place within the HSE, the role of the Department, and the recent creation of a nursing unit within the HR division of the HSE. They also saw a need to agree on what role, if any, nursing advisors should have within this structure.

A Delphi study for WHO Europe[245] identified the ideal attributes of a chief nurse as communication, teamworking, strategic thinking, professional credibility, leadership, political astuteness, decency and integrity, innovation, decision-making and problem-solving, personal qualities, promotion of nursing, good management and conflict resolution, information handling, research skills and physical characteristics. The study was conducted as part of an initiative to advance the role of the chief nurse in member countries of the WHO in Europe. It concluded that, in order to advance the role, it was necessary to engage in a systematic selection and recruitment of suitable post holders and introduce a critical pathway for development of both new recruits and existing personnel.

There was a broader concern among interviewees about the level of clinical representation at the highest level within the HSE. It so happens that the current chief executive of the HSE is a clinical person, but, as an educator observed, there are no provisions with the structures that are envisaged within the *Prospectus Report* for a clinical person at the highest level. Some spoke about the need for a clinical voice at the top decision-making table and regretted that it was not a requirement in the new structures.

A number of interviewees said that it was difficult to identify nurse managers who were capable of moving beyond the bounds of nursing itself and taking on board the broader demands of executive functions across the whole hospital. There were some good examples of this, but not enough, and it was often a question of preparing them for that role, a preparation that did not exist at the moment.

One service manager spoke about the need for directors of nursing to consider their broader corporate presence within the organisation:

> When I look at a director of nursing, she is the director of nursing but when you are directing a hospital like this, you really are a senior executive of a hospital at a board level and at every level.

There was an idea of an 'executive nurse' rather than just a 'director of nursing' that says something about the wider role that nursing needs to have within the services:

> Director of NMPDU: To me, it is about moving to a situation whereby we develop executive nurses rather than directors of nursing and it is that executive leadership that nurses must become more proactively involved in.

It was not enough that nurse managers were good at managing nursing; they needed to be able to expand beyond the borders of the professions to present the nursing voice at the wider executive table:

> Educator: They can perform very effectively in their own arena and I would suggest that their own arena does not provide enough of a challenge for them once they get to that point. I think we need to face some of our nurse leaders with the fact that that simply is not enough; it is not what you are doing your MBA for. It is not what you are doing your doctorate for. It is not why you get to be director of nursing in the big large teaching hospitals. You are there because you have to be sufficiently confident to know that you can perform well beyond that arena.

This failure to reach out beyond the immediate boundaries of nursing may be due to an in-built culture of passivity within the professions that needs to be named and tackled.

Ultimately, according to interviewees, this was about positioning directors of nursing within the decision-making structures in the services. It differed from one hospital to another and from one setting to another, but it was an integral part of the clinicians in management approach that was being developed within the HSE and that, in turn, would build on the clinicians in management initiative that has been developed over the last number of years.

The directors of nursing spoke about the difficulty of making the voice of nursing heard at the decision-making table within the executive structure in the hospital and said that they needed to be involved in shaping the services of the future; otherwise they would be left behind. This would mean positioning the role of the director of nursing more clearly within the system and ensuring that reporting relationships and duties were clearly understood. One service manager mentioned a director of nursing being asked to report to a much lower administrative grade and said that this was not unique. However, directors of nursing were very clear about the ability, competence and levels of education that existed within their group to enable them to take their place at the table. They said that nurses were a very experienced, versatile and, increasingly, well-educated group, with many now possessing postgraduate qualifications in a wide range of management disciplines:

> Director of nursing and midwifery: We need to get that recognised in some way in this new structure… and get those nurses into the different change management teams that will be out there leading the change.

They noted the difficulty that many institutions were experiencing in recruiting senior nurse managers. This was leaving significant gaps at senior level within the professions and was evidence of unwillingness to take on these challenges. One director of an NMPDU suggested the introduction of mentoring services to advance the leaders of the future. Nursing was not seen as investing in its own future, mentoring and bringing on the next batch of senior managers, because of its preoccupation with micro-management of services, and it was not surprising, therefore, that people were not applying for senior posts as they become vacant. Other NMPDU directors also mentioned this.

This group said that, as newer opportunities had emerged because of the opening up of a wider range of career pathways, there were more and more attractive clinical options open to nurses and midwives. It had always been the complaint of nurses and midwives that the only paths forward for them lay in either management or education. This was no longer the case and was a nurse management challenge that had not been foreseen.

Nurse educators also voiced this opinion. Said one: 'I am concerned that people are not competing for those very senior posts, that there really are issues about bringing people into management'. The nurse educators felt that the role was not seen as attractive and that the problem was also related to a lack of identity for the grade of nurse management below that of director of nursing. People at assistant director of nursing level had a crisis of identity about their role and their future:

> Educator: It is disappointing to hear young, very energised, very well-educated assistant directors wanting out of their jobs and asking you, 'where are the opportunities or should I go for this or should I go for that?' Which you could see as being a sideline move, but they are not seeing applying for the top job as being as attractive as it should be.

This raised the important question about support for nurse managers, nurse leaders of management development and succession planning within the professions and, in particular, within the management structures of the professions.

Nurse-/Midwife-Led Services

The role of the nurse and midwife as coordinator of both clinical and management/logistics services within the clinical setting was

Table 17: Research Issues: Nurse-/Midwife-Led Services

Theme	Frequency of mention
It is important that the coordinating role of nurses and midwives in clinical settings is understood and appreciated more	14
There will be an increase in the amount of nurse-/midwife-led clinical services	56

highlighted by a good number of interviewees without any prompting by the interviewer. The coordinating role of nurses and midwives and increased nurse-/midwife-led clinical services were the two themes discussed (see Table 17).

Nurse-/midwife-led care is provided by nurses and midwives responsible for case management, which includes comprehensive patient/client assessment, developing, implementing and managing a plan of care, clinical leadership and a decision to admit or discharge. Such care requires enhanced skills and knowledge and the nurse will need preparation in both the clinical and management aspects of the role. Such nurses will be practising at an advanced level and may be working in approved specialist or advanced practice roles.

One simple statement encapsulated the views of most:

> Educator: I think nurses have a lot of skills and are eminently good coordinators. They spend at least 50 per cent of their time coordinating. They spend an awful lot of their time liaising with other people.

Others referred to the fact that, within clinical settings, nurses were there all the time. Doctors, physiotherapists, occupational therapists, dieticians and other service providers came and went, but nurses provided a 24/7 service. The shift system, and the 'unit nursing officer'/ward sister/CNM role made them eminently suitable for this role of coordinating the inputs and services of all other service providers. They were also intimately involved in managing the logistics of the clinical setting and were, therefore, well suited to a broader general management role within the setting. One service manager expressed this in an interesting way:

> They are kind of the glue and I am just a bit worried that… because there is such specialisation, they may not be the glue anymore.

Other interviewees voiced the concern that the move towards increased specialisation of roles within nursing and midwifery, with CNSs/CMSs and ANPs/AMPs, could detract from this overall coordinating role of the nurse. The earlier discussion about clinical career pathways addressed some of these concerns and emphasised the need for continued support for the generalist role of the nurse, as someone within the clinical area who knows who to call in when a crisis arises.

This coordinating role however was seen as particularly important when one looked at the role of the ward sister or CNM2:

> Director of NMPDU: They are strong on things like clinical audit and teamwork. You look at ward sisters and their main role is to coordinate the functions on a medical or surgical ward, so they are used to dealing with the different disciplines. I would see the CNM2s as being the most skilled people on wards because they organise care.

What emerged from comments such as this is the concept of the general nurse/midwife, and, in particular, the unit/ward manager – ward sister, CNM2 – as the coordinator of a wide range of services within the clinical setting and the organiser of care. This is a role that requires a complex range of skills and understanding and the ability to deal with all of the disciplines. It is a vision of nursing that permeated many comments and was to be found underlying other comments on a wide range of topics. It is, therefore, a central concept, something that is distinct from the role of the specialist nurse, and one that is eminently complemented by the specialist role. Specialist nurses are in a position to provide wide-ranging support to general nurses in clinical areas along with the many other advantages already discussed.

The concept of nurses and midwives as coordinators of services, and the emergence of increased specialisation of services, led on to the idea of nurse-/midwife-led services, a topic that attracted many comments. There was agreement that a major increase in the amount and variety of nurse-/midwife-led services in the future was inevitable and desirable.

Medical consultants showed no hesitation in advocating an increase in the range of nurse-/midwife-led services. There was frequent reference to the importance of the work of the National Council in facilitating and encouraging the development of CNS/CMS and ANP/AMP roles within frameworks of practice.

A number of interviewees said that midwifery had played a lead role in the provision of nurse-/midwife-led services. The following comment from a medical consultant sums up the views of many:

> Already in this institution, for example, we have set up a home birth service which is run totally by the midwives and, indeed, we have had directly led midwifery services and midwife clinics now for 20 years.

One medical consultant referred to the idea of 'devolvement of normal healthy pregnant women to midwives'. A number of interviewees raised the general idea of referrals to nurses and midwives as a feature of nurse-/midwife-led services, something that appeared to be particularly attractive in both primary and acute settings for a wide range of health issues and across all of the divisions of nursing.

The idea of nurses acting autonomously within primary care settings, taking referrals from GPs and referring on to medical consultants and other professionals where necessary, or acute services generally, is one that sat quite comfortably with interviewees. One NMPDU director spoke of the emergence of 'a general nurse practitioner in the same way that you have a general practitioner in medicine. They would have their own clinics; they would have their own surgeries; they would have their own service day units; and so on'.

Nurse-/midwife-led services are discussed in the next two sections, on interdisciplinary teams and the development of relationships between primary and acute care settings. It is not a new concept in health care.

Interdisciplinary Teams

The desirability of nurses to work as part of interdisciplinary teams was a topic that came up under a number of different themes and categories. This has been noted in the sections on clinical career pathways, leadership and nurse-/midwife-led services. All interviewees who commented on this topic (Table 18)

Table 18: Research Issues: Interdisciplinary Teams

Theme	Frequency of mention
There will be an increased involvement of nurses and midwives in interdisciplinary teams	54

were agreed that it was both desirable and inevitable that nurses and midwives would find themselves in the future working more and more in multidisciplinary and interdisciplinary teams.

Many comments centred on the importance of nursing developing the confidence to participate in these teams and to assert the nursing voice as an equal member of the team. Many also said that there was still a lack of confidence in this area:

> Service manager: It's getting better but they almost felt they had to be spoken to rather than speaking out themselves and they didn't see themselves as equal, even within the multidisciplinary teams.

Nursing, through education and practice, was seen as becoming more self-confident. It is seen, to quote one service manager, as emerging as the profession that is 'with the client', 'at the front line and in touch with the realities of patients and clients' needs', and 'in possession of the necessary skills to assess and address these needs'. Many mentioned the value of education in increasing this confidence and ability to take part as an equal in these teams. In acute settings involved in the hospital accreditation process, another service manager commented: 'where you are seeing the change is in places with the accreditation where there are multidisciplinary teams. The nursing voice is starting to rise'.

The likelihood of nurses and midwives providing a wider range of nursing-/midwifery-led services in primary settings usually drew comments about the importance of multidisciplinary teamworking. The reality of multidisciplinary working was seen as a natural corollary of providing more nurse-/midwife-led services.

Interviewees commented that nursing should not see itself as the 'Cinderella' of the multidisciplinary team but as having a vital and central role to play in it. There were comments from nurse leaders that they had a responsibility to go out and promote this concept:

> Director of NMPDU: There is an onus on us all as nurse leaders to go out there and support mechanisms to help that to happen.

This need to promote the role of nursing within the team was related to the fact that, traditionally, medical consultants have seen themselves as the natural leaders of the interdisciplinary team. Interviewees saw this as changing over time, but it would require a change of culture, something that would be greatly helped by changes in the education and training of nurses over time. However, nurses would need to move outside of their traditional comfort zone:

> Service manager: I see a problem of nurse leadership in leading other professions. I think they can lead within their own discipline but they can feel out of their own comfort zone when it is with other disciplines, so I think now, with better education, they can take an equal place at the table.

Medical consultants recognised that the challenge of interdisciplinarity was not an easy one, as professionals, including nurses, were becoming more assertive in their own disciplines.

Relationship between Primary and Acute Care Services

The wider question of relations between primary and acute settings was discussed in relation to organisational changes within the health services of the future, about systems pressure within future health services, and in a number of other areas. It is, therefore, a central issue within this research. It is of particular relevance to the transformation programme that is at the core of the development priorities of the HSE (see Table 19).

Table 19: Research Issues: Relationship between Primary and Acute Services

Theme	Frequency of mention
Nurses from acute services will most likely get involved in follow-through services to clients in the community on their discharge from the acute services	12
There is likely to be an increase in the numbers of nurses and midwives active in the community	33

In 2006, the National Council published a report entitled *Improving the Patient Journey: Understanding Integrated Care Pathways.*[246] This emphasised the importance of integrated care pathways and provided guidance for nurses and midwives in implementing integrated care pathways. An essential feature is the development of partnership and collaboration arrangements with interdisciplinary teams across the continuum of care facilities.

There is evidence in the research undertaken for this book that there is a commitment, both at the policy level and at the executive level, to build the services of the future around this central concept of a shift from acute to primary care services. It is also clear that nursing and midwifery will have a central role to play in this. The policy commitment is to the development in areas across the board. Some interviewees quoted international best practice in this area. For example, one policymaker said:

> I understand that in Paris there are over a thousand hospital nurses who work in the community on early discharge arrangements and I would like to see something like that happening in Dublin.

The approach was frequently associated with managing occupancy rates and early discharges that are made more feasible when nurses and midwives follow through with direct support to patients/clients in their own community settings. This was seen as not without its difficulties, as the issue of industrial relations and the cooperation of the unions was not underestimated. As another policymaker noted, 'they can contribute hugely in the community if we can get around the logistical and IR [industrial relations] issues. But that is going to take time'.

Trade union interviewees spoke of their commitment to the value of this approach, referring to the value it had in terms of job satisfaction and in the value it brought to the quality of patient care. However, according to one service manager, the experience of the recent NAMIC (nursing and midwifery in the community) initiative suggested that, in practice, there was a lot of union opposition to the changes required to make it happen. Within service management, the commitment was explicit:

> Service manager: The first change we are going to see is that services are going to be moved out of hospitals so there is no point in nurses and doctors being left in hospitals to the degree that they are at present. They have got to follow where the patients are.

Service managers said that nurses and midwives had a clear role in this shift from acute to primary and in the creation of bridges between the two sides of the services. Indeed the expectation and the hope was that nurses and midwives should lead this shift. One service manager commented that this might have implications for the configuration of local hospital services as 'that means our local hospital may only have GPs and ANPs. Now you could turn that on its head and say your local hospital will be much better off than it is at the moment'.

It was, therefore, expected that the quality of service provided at a local level should be substantially enhanced by this approach. An important dimension was empowering patients/clients to take responsibility for their own needs within their own setting. This was particularly true for people with chronic conditions, such as diabetes:

> Director of NMPDU: So much could be done to have people with those conditions nursed at home and I don't even want to emphasise 'nursed' but rather 'empowered' to manage their own conditions almost in a very proactive way in the environment that they wish.

It is not possible to talk about nursing in the community without talking about the role of the PHN, a role that came in for a good deal of criticism within this research. Interviewees felt that the role was not well defined, either as a generalist role or as a specialist role, and that it was not clear what development priorities had been identified for it. There was also criticism for the way in which the role of the PHN has been managed, with evidence of a considerable amount of resistance to change not being tackled by management.

Some also referred to an increasing fragmentation in the way in which nursing and midwifery services were delivered within the community, with no clear definition of the relative complementary nature of the roles of the staff nurse, the PHN and the other grades of CNSs, ANPs and midwives in the community. One educator commented that the role of the PHN should become more policy- and education-focused, with more specialist nurses in the community supporting that role.

This suggestion is perhaps more in line with what was envisaged for this role by the Commission on Nursing, which saw the role of the director of public health nursing as a mirror within the community of the role of the director of nursing within the acute sector. Both roles were intended by the Commission to be more strategic in nature, providing leadership to other grades of nursing.

The reality is that much is happening in primary care without any direct involvement of PHNs. Their role, said interviewees, would, therefore, come under increased scrutiny as to their relevance:

> Service manager: If the profession is to survive in primary care, in particular, nurses will have to demonstrate that what they are doing is viable, that it is visible and is credible and I think that it won't be. I mean, the public health nurses are a classic example at the moment. Primary care is developing without them so you have to ask: is what they are doing viable and credible and is it visible?

In 2006 a report[247] by the School of Nursing, Dublin City University, focused on identifying the core elements of nursing care deemed important for community-registered general nurses. The report said that there were 430 nurses in the INO database, whose primary role was to support the PHN in community care in Ireland The report states that the Commission on Nursing had already raised concerns about the integration of the diverse range of nursing groups providing nursing services in the community and had stated that 'there is a need for the profession to develop a coherent vision for the future direction of nursing in the community which reflects the nursing needs of the community rather than the status of individual groups within the profession'. This was the first substantial study on the role of the registered general nurse working in the community within Irish health care.

Conclusions

Based on the primary research that has been conducted in this chapter, and on the research outlined in the earlier chapters of this book, it is possible to identify key elements of the future role of nursing and midwifery in Ireland as perceived by the stakeholders who took part in the research.

An overarching message about the role is one of integration across the professions and a recognition that it is important to break down barriers between management, education, clinical practice, research and professional development. For that reason, in considering the future role and in identifying the elements that will be part of that role, an integrated approach is adopted. This involves looking at the overall professions and considering the constituent parts of the professions as mutually complementary and reinforcing, and dispensing with any indication of hierarchical relationships between the various parts. This is a theme that will be returned to when we consider the strategy for the professional development of nursing and midwifery. With this in mind, the following points represent a summary of the key findings of the research in relation to the future role of nursing and midwifery:

- It is time to review the rationale for maintaining five points of entry to the professions. The demands of the service and of patients and clients for increased integration and interdisciplinarity point to the need for the application of these principles to the way in which nurses and midwives are educated.
- A clinical career pathway should continue to exist and evolve in line with service and professional needs. This should define levels of practice. The levels of practice should include:
  - General nurse/midwife
  - CNS and CMS
  - ANP and AMP.
- A management career pathway should continue to exist and evolve in line with service and professional needs. This pathway should change and adapt to service development requirements. It should include:
  - Frontline management, i.e. clinical nurse managers with a grading structure that matches the context of service delivery
  - Middle management, i.e. assistant directors of nursing and divisional nurse managers, in accordance with the requirements of the service delivery context
  - Senior management, i.e. directors of nursing.
- Opportunities for the development of career pathways in other areas (education, research and professional development) should also be explored in order to provide a richer range of career options for nurses and midwives.
- Nursing and midwifery should operate on the basis of a primary/acute care continuum – nurses and midwives should move seamlessly between acute and primary care settings in line with the needs of the patients. The modalities of this should be agreed with health service managers and should be conducted in accordance with agreed protocols.
- Nurses and midwives should play an active role in primary care teams. This should include, where necessary, acting as

leader of the team or as a member of the team with other professionals.

- As part of their role within the primary/acute care continuum nurses and midwives should continue to develop nurse-/ midwife-led clinical services. These services should be developed in consultation with health service managers and should reflect the levels of practice and the career pathway of the individual nurse or midwife. It should include as appropriate:
  - Management of case loads in both acute and community settings in accordance with agreed practice protocols and in line with their levels of practice
  - Management of early discharge from acute settings and follow up with the patient/client in the community, including, where appropriate, in their own home
  - Diagnosis of conditions in accordance with agreed practice protocols
  - Treating and prescribing in accordance with agreed practice protocols
  - Referring clients/patients to other areas of service delivery and other professionals in accordance with the needs of the patient/client
  - Taking referrals from other areas of the services and from other professionals in accordance with the needs of the patient/client
  - Education and empowerment of patients/clients in the community settings and in their own homes in the management of their own health.
- Nurses and midwives should prescribe medications in accordance with the provisions of legislation and after having completed the required education and training programmes and achieved registration as a registered nurse prescriber/ registered midwife prescriber with An Bord Altranais.
- Nurses and midwives should act as members and, where appropriate, as leaders of interdisciplinary and multidisciplinary teams within acute and primary care settings.
- Nurses and midwives should incorporate the roles of health care assistants, home helps and other support staff into the delivery of their services as appropriate in both acute and

primary care services, and in line with agreed protocols and practice.

- Nurses and midwives should continue to develop relationships with medical consultants, doctors and other health care professionals that reflect the development of their roles within their career pathways and in line with service needs. This should include identification of complementarity, development of an understanding of what each professional can bring to a multidisciplinary team, breaking down silos of practice and encouraging a culture of common decision-making, collaborative working and multidisciplinary service delivery.
- In acute care settings, nurse and midwife managers should have an input into areas of service management that affect the delivery of nursing and midwifery services. This should include involvement in bed management, where the role of nurses and midwives and their broad knowledge and understanding of the services equip them to play a distinctive role. It should also include involvement in quality development initiatives where nurses and midwives have frequently taken a lead role. In addition, it should include, where appropriate, control of and management of services of hygiene, laundry, catering and other logistical activities that affect the total quality of care for the patient/client in the acute care setting. The involvement of nurses and midwives in these areas should be agreed in accordance with management protocols developed at the local level in accordance with service and professional development needs.
- Nurses and midwives should play an active role in engaging with the clinicians in a leadership initiative. This initiative should build on the experience of models for the involvement of clinicians in management and leadership that have evolved in different care settings and should take account of the experience that has been developed through these models. Nurses and midwives should cooperate as part of a clinical management team, as either active members or as leaders, depending on service and professional needs.
- Nurses and midwives should play meaningful roles in both the strategic planning of health services within the HSE and the development of policies and performance management

protocols within the Department of Health and Children. This should require nurses and midwives to demonstrate that they possess the competencies that are required to make a meaningful contribution at this level. It should also require the HSE and the Department to facilitate the involvement of competent nurses and midwives in this role.

- The importance of the clinical voice at national level should be examined by the HSE, with a view to ensuring that, at the level of national director within the services, this is guaranteed.
- Nurses and midwives should explore with HSE management innovative approaches to the resolution of disputes without the need to have recourse to industrial action. This should involve maximum use of the partnership mechanisms that are already in place. Nurse and midwife staff associations and trade unions should continue to fulfil a key role on behalf of the professions within these partnership structures and as advocates of general conditions for nurses and midwives. The resolution of disputes should be conducted on the basis of respect for all parties to the dispute and for the role of nursing and midwife managers at local and regional level.
- Nurses and midwives should incorporate the use of ICT into their practice within each of the career pathways, in accordance with service and professional needs.
- The role of nurses and midwives should expand in line with agreed frameworks for scope of practice. This should include a dynamic evolution of the role in line with service needs and professional development.
- The role of nurses and midwives should evolve and develop in line with demographic and epidemiological trends and should respond to the need for change in a proactive way, providing leadership within the professions in adapting to the needs of patients and clients within the services.

The next chapter in this research will explore the challenges of building the necessary skills and competencies that will be required to fulfil this role in the future health services.

CHAPTER 10

Research Results: Building Skills and Competencies

In the third and final part of the research, those interviewed were asked to discuss five questions relating to the skills and competencies required by nurses and midwives in the changing health services and the education provisions designed to provide them with the necessary academic support in attaining and maintaining those skills. The questions were as follows:

- What do you think are the key skills and competencies that nurses and midwives will need to develop to fulfil their role within the future health services?
- In what way do these new skills differ from the present range of skills?
- Do you believe that, on the whole, nurses and midwives already have these skills?
- How would you assess the appropriateness of the current range of educational provisions for nurses and midwives in view of the changes ahead?
- What changes would you suggest in the provision of education and training for nurses and midwives?

The responses of interviewees are examined under eight thematic headings:

1. Current skill levels
2. Differences from future skills requirements
3. Future skills required
4. Skill mix
5. Pre-registration education
6. Post-registration education
7. Continuing professional development
8. Common education.

Current Skill Levels

There were two predominant comments on the current skill levels of nurses and midwives, shown in Table 20. Most interviewees disagreed with the statement that nurses and midwives currently possessed the skills to face the future challenges of a changing health service. Despite this negative message, the overall tone of respondents to the levels of skills in nursing and midwifery was not negative. Many were very positive and most recognised that things were changing fast and that everybody, not just nurses and midwives, had a lot of work to do to adapt and learn what was needed.

Table 20: Research Issues: Current Skill Levels

Theme	Frequency of mention
Nurses and midwives currently possess the necessary skills to face the future challenges of a changing health service	29
A change in the skill levels of a small number of nurses and midwives can have a significant impact on the quality of care provided in a clinical setting	36

90 per cent agreed that a change in skill levels of a small number of nurses and midwives could have a major impact on the quality of care provided in a clinical setting. This refers to what may be loosely described as the 'bell curve' phenomenon, i.e. shifting some members of the group to the right of the probability distribution curve for skill levels within a clinical setting, resulting in a shift of the curve and a dramatic improvement in skill levels and in quality and safety. (The use of the term 'bell curve' in this context is not intended to have any statistical validity in terms of distribution patterns of skill levels but simply to illustrate the impact of changes within a group.)

A policymaker interviewee suggested the idea:

> I suppose that any group of people's skills are probably distributed according to the bell shape curve and you've got the vast majority of people in the middle. The whole thrust of what we should be doing now in terms of the reform programme is simply to move the bell curve to the right so that if you get a little bit of improvement in all of these people, things improve dramatically.

A number of participants spoke about the impact that education and training could have on the overall level of skills and on the quality of care that was delivered in a clinical setting. One service manager, who felt that nurses and midwives in general did not possess the skills to equip them for the challenges of the future, referred to the importance of constantly assessing and evaluating the roles of nurses and midwives within the clinical setting as a complement to what was done in education and training. This idea of 'looking at your own role' – critically assessing and evaluating your own role – is something that was perceived by this participant as a new and welcome phenomenon in nursing and midwifery, something that had not been happening in the past:

> Service manager: No they don't have them but we are getting there, through education and the fact that they have looked at their own role; but they have got to more critically look at it all the time on an evolving basis, and that's what they weren't doing. You have to constantly look, and we all have to look at our roles.

Some spoke about the impact that education was having on the professions, but also pointed out that there was still a very large cohort of nurses and midwives who were in the system for a long time and had very little development. These represented the large bulk of nurses and midwives who 'gravitate towards hands-on patient concerns', according to a service manager, who 'focus on individual patients and individual clinical skills', suggested a regulator, and who 'have worked in county hospitals... busy taking care of the elderly and haven't got the time off', said an educator.

Interviewees praised the work that the National Council, the NMPDUs and the CNEs were doing, but spoke about the need for wide-scale interventions to make a greater impact and about the need for nursing and midwifery to be, according to a service manager, more 'aggressive in forcing training and demanding time and locums for people to be developed and skilled'.

They spoke about the need to build an understanding that we are moving away from a delivery system that, said a regulator, 'focuses on individual patients and individual clinical skills to a community-based or family-based set of skills' and that these skills were emerging and were beginning to be developed well.

One service manager expressed this idea:

> These skills need to be nurtured more, and I think there needs to be a realisation that we are moving away from an autonomous delivery to a more collaborative approach in terms of service delivery and that is where our challenge will be.

This meant that, as an educator put it, 'the hierarchical system may have been diluted', and managers and clinicians 'have different relationships with each other and with the people that they are managing', but that 'it is still hard for people to step outside of that because it takes a long time'. This idea of a new set of relationships between everybody involved in service management and service delivery emerged as a key characteristic of the services of the future and, therefore, a key determinant of the skill sets required.

Other interviewees spoke about the need to learn by exposure to good practice, by experiencing what it felt like – for example, to work in a multidisciplinary team environment:

> Service manager: I believe they don't actually understand what it means and, in fact, the only way to educate people ultimately may be to arrange placements of students into teams that function well even for a week or two. Because I think that unless you actually see how a multidisciplinary team works well, you can't actually understand it.

In all of this, there was a core idea of the need for linkages between the clinical setting and education providers, including all those involved in the planning, accreditation, delivery and financing of professional development, continuing professional development and in-service education. Building skills for the future, building an understanding of what was needed for the future, and making an impact on a large cohort of nurses and midwives within the professions would be a collaborative venture across a range of different stakeholders and institutional settings.

Differences from Future Skills Requirements

Asked how the skills needed for the future differed from the present range of skills, there were two main areas of comment (see Table 21). All interviewees agreed that there was a difference between the levels of skills required now and those that would be required in the future and that there was a need for continuity with the present, coupled with the ability to prepare for and adapt to change.

Table 21: Research Issues: Differences from Future Skills Requirements

Theme	Frequency of mention
There is a need for continuity with the present, coupled with the ability to prepare for and adapt to change	48
There are some specific skills that will be needed in the future	77

When expressing themselves about the difference between the skills of today and those of the future, interviewees frequently used terms like 'taking more responsibility', 'being more accountable', 'more autonomy' and 'more decision-making'. They also believed that there would be more multidisciplinary and interdisciplinary working, and more community-based services, with consequent implications for educational and training programmes. Another topic that came up very frequently was confidence – the importance of nursing and midwifery having the confidence to take its place as an equal member of the team, to lead the team where needed, to articulate its opinion and to ensure that it was heard.

The growing importance of primary care in the health services of the future has featured throughout all of this research. It was voiced by an educator in the context of the skills and competencies needed for the future and the implications this had for the kind of programmes developed:

> We are producing nurses now and, in five to ten years time, 80 per cent or 75 per cent of them, in fact, are going to be in community roles. Our educational focus should be shifting to take that into account.

This meant breaking down what was referred to on a number of occasions as 'the silo approach' to service delivery, moving towards a more outward-looking interdisciplinary approach and, as a policymaker phrased it, 'a willingness to take on board the attitudes and the skills that are necessary to accommodate that way of doing work'. This, along with the importance of a shift to primary care and community-based services, were two key mantras.

Interviewees spoke about the new role being 'more proactive, with a greater degree of autonomy, which will also bring with it increased expectations'. One educator said that the current role 'is very much about delivering and doing. I think the next generation of nursing… is about leading, about autonomous practice'. This implied taking on more responsibility, particularly, for example, in the area of nurse-/midwife-led clinics and in leading teams of service delivery. A service manager said that the implication of this was that nurses and midwives would need a more rounded education and training for that role, one that encompassed training in skills that had not traditionally been part of the nursing and midwifery education curriculum.

Some referred to the potential for nursing and midwifery to occupy a central role in managing caseloads and case teams because of the versatility and flexibility of their experience. Medical consultants believed that nurses and midwives were ideally placed because of the breadth of their role. Many other roles within the clinical area (e.g. physiotherapists, occupational therapists and dieticians) had a very narrow focus, whereas nursing took on a greater degree of ownership of the overall clinical situation.

Related to this was the concept of the nurse in the community being able to develop relationships with patients and clients to educate them and to empower them to manage their own health. One educator commented that this required the credibility 'to educate, negotiate, bargain and work with people in a way that no other professional can do'. This encouraged a much more proactive approach from nursing and this would become even more pronounced with the introduction of nurse prescribing. It was a new way of working for nursing:

> Service manager: I think that in some ways nursing will be the decision-making final port of call but with a lot of ANPs and not having to have decisions signed off by other therapists or doctors.

Many interviewees spoke of the need for nursing and midwifery to develop more confidence rather than more competence. They felt that the educational system that had been put in place, and the opportunities for professional development that had been developed since the Commission on Nursing, were envied by many other countries and would produce very competent nurses. According to one educator:

> In many ways, we are the envy of a number of countries; we are the envy of the United States and we are the envy of parts of the UK in actually getting our degree programme. So we have come a long way in a very short time, after a long period of pretty much not a lot. I think the Commission has done a lot in terms of a blueprint and ideas for the future, etc., but if we are going to move this profession, we have got to stand up and be counted and be willing to take the rough with the smooth, not hiding behind whoever it is and feeling that it is nice to have someone else to blame when it does not happen.

As the hierarchical nature of the health services changed radically, one medical consultant commented:

> The power base is shifting and we are becoming more and more advocates, advisors, facilitators and less and less are we in a power relationship. That is calling for different skills: advisory skills, communications skills. It is calling for people to be better able to explain their judgements and their decisions.

A number of interviewees referred to a study[248] carried out in 2000 on behalf of the Office for Health Management, which listed the competencies that would be required by senior nurse and midwife managers and which provided a useful point of reference when considering the competencies and skills that will be needed in the present and future.

Future Skills Required

What skills and competencies will nurses and midwives require in the future? Seven main areas are cited in Table 22. There was full agreement about the need for these skills, with the exception of financial skills, for which there was 90 per cent agreement. Quite a number spoke about the complementary nature of many of the skills and spoke more about the kind of person that was needed – well rounded, broadly educated, and with a strong sense of professional identity and accountability.

This gives us an opportunity to take a closer look at some of the more specific skills that interviewees chose to highlight as being of importance to the future role of nurses and midwives in the health services. One interviewee from education spoke about 'a fundamental skill, a human interaction skill'. Included in this was

Table 22: Research Issues: Future Skills Required

Theme	Frequency of mention
Nurses and midwives will need communications skills	47
Nurses and midwives will need greater understanding of, and training in, financial skills for healthcare professionals	48
The ability to work in an interdisciplinary environment will be an important dimension of the future skills required of nurses and midwives	32
Management skills will be very important for nurses and midwives	24
People management skills will be very important for nurses and midwives	44
Nurses and midwives will need more highly developed research skills	49
Nurses and midwives will be more specialised in future health services	13

the idea of respect for persons, colleagues, patients and clients. This 'fundamental skill' provided a platform, a context on which to build skills like communication, working in teams, interdisciplinarity, people management and general management. It also provided the basis for an ability to speak out courageously on issues that were important. It provided the basis for the self-confidence that nurses and midwives would need to intervene and make their voices heard in public debates and private discussions on how the services should be developed and delivered, and on issues of importance to staff and patients.

Many interviewees highlighted people management as a problem within nursing:

> Service manager: We have seen a lot of problems in relation to people management within nursing. Management have to intervene a lot more than they should have to in people management areas within nursing.

A number said that there continued to be a lot of bullying and destructive behaviour within the profession of nursing. One reference was made to a quality of life survey conducted among health services staff in a wide geographic area that showed that bullying was most prevalent in nursing. Most of the bullying came from within the profession, it was claimed, but also from patients and from across the disciplines of medicine and administration.

The main problem, according to the survey, appeared to be how nurses and midwives felt they were being managed or disempowered within their own professions. Interviewees spoke about individual nurses and midwives feeling that they were being 'got at' by their nurse managers, that the interpretation of rules was being used in a very unfair way to individuals at ward level. The problem also existed at more senior levels within nursing and midwifery. Interviewees also spoke about the problem of a director of nursing's span of control being too wide to enable him or her to detect problems such as these at lower levels within the system.

Part of the problem, according to a number of interviewees, was that people were expected to slot immediately into management roles without any adequate preparation, without serious thought being given to the 'people management' skills and the support managers needed:

> Service manager: People management is the most difficult bit of management… it is the subtlety in how you manage people. And it is not fair to ask somebody on day one to supervise maybe ten or twenty of their colleagues without them having had an opportunity to work through the skills that are involved in that.

Bullying and treating colleagues badly stem from a lack of fundamental communication skills in such areas as interaction, showing sympathy, people management and handling stressful situations. The latter was deemed to be an essential skill in situations involving 'either a vulnerable public or a demanding public' – typical situations for nurses and midwives to deal with. One educator referred to the 'gentleness required with our own staff and with patients, particularly in difficult situations'. This was particularly important in determining the borderline between being 'assertive' and being 'aggressive'. Knowing the difference and being aware of how one came across was a skill and a level of awareness that was frequently lacking in nursing and midwifery:

> Service manager: I don't think we do half enough in terms of training our future managers of any kind in the health services. It is all hit and miss and grabbing the odd course here and relying on people's own skills, but compared to the NHS we are still not at the races.

The view was expressed that this involved a complex set of competencies in human interaction rather than a list of self-contained, isolated skills. What was required was an approach to developing the whole person. Much of this could be achieved through education and personal development, which implied that there was a need to take a critical look at the pre- and post-registration nursing and midwifery education programmes.

Concern was expressed about the 'ability to destroy' people that existed within the professions, and the lack of insight and self-awareness that perpetrators of such behaviour might have had. While it was acknowledged that this 'destructive force' needed to be contained, one interviewee claimed that there were situations where individual nurses and midwives experienced considerable resistance from senior managers when they sought to improve themselves through education and training. People were being blocked from becoming specialists or ANPs and AMPs in their areas and being forced to give up their jobs to take on further education. This was described by an educator as 'some pockets of unbelievable resistance and ignorance and lack of willingness to support staff in the system, particularly in the acute hospital sector, I would say they are not desperately very visible'.

The 'destructive force' is latent but potent. One policymaker described this in graphic terms: 'Nurses are not always kind to one another as people managers… they crucify one another'. Nevertheless, few suggestions for dealing with this culture of destructiveness were forthcoming. One of the educators commented that if nursing and midwifery could dissipate the most destructive elements within the professions,

> … then I would say we are well on the way. I think we certainly have the capacity. I think there is awareness, but also a fear. The fear can be somehow dissipated partially by getting more information into the system and not being afraid to say you do not have the information.

This interviewee went on to say that nurses and midwives needed to be prepared to challenge each other at every level in a positive and constructive way. This meant asking a lot more questions, and doing a lot more thinking about staff support, and encouraging staff to talk to each other, to share their uncertainties, and helping them to live with those uncertainties.

One service manager spoke about the difficulty in recruiting directors of nursing and midwifery with an appropriate level of management competence. This difficulty arose from the narrow experience base of many of the candidates and the fact that there were not enough people coming through the system with the required level of management competence. Another service manager commented that an MBA (master of business administration) was valuable but not sufficient to prepare someone to manage up to a thousand staff in a large acute tertiary referral hospital. Their narrow experience base, together with their insufficient level of management skill, presented challenges for the training and education of senior managers within nursing and midwifery. This was in contrast to what many participants referred to as the broad-based competence of nurses and midwives in clinical settings and their overall understanding of hospitals and the health system.

It is particularly exacerbated in what one referred to as 'the paralysed environment' that had emerged within some large acute hospitals because of bitter industrial relations disputes. It was unfair to expect someone to move up to a senior post in such circumstances and expect them to manage without adequate preparation and training.

Interviewees also spoke about other areas of management that should be included in a list of competencies:

> Service manager: Empowering patients, problem-solving, project management focus, engagement with partnership, reflection, quality assurance audit, evidence-based protocols and guidelines, and what I call real accountable management, like appraisal and dealing with IR and giving and taking feedback and leadership.

With regard to specialisation, one director of nursing and midwifery expressed reservations about the possible exploitation of CNSs/CMSs and ANPs/AMPs by other disciplines, saying that every medical consultant in the hospital was looking for CNSs. She also warned of the danger of becoming dependent on one individual. For example, an ANP would build up a reputable and valuable clinical practice within the hospital, but problems would occur within the service if the post-holder went on extended leave and no replacement was put in place. Other members of the focus group did not support this view, which illustrates a not unhealthy lack of consensus among senior nurse managers of acute hospitals in relation to the increased specialisation of nurses and midwives, and the role they could play within acute, specialised and community hospital settings. Within the same group, others spoke in glowing terms about the roles they could play and about the need to ensure that they also had the opportunity to follow up their patients into the community.

Interviewees mentioned the importance of building within nursing and midwifery a research competence to underpin the increased emphasis on evidence-based practice. They spoke about the need to educate nurses and midwives in research skills and to examine opportunities for increased involvement of nurses and midwives in dedicated research activities. A service manager suggested the development of opportunities within nursing and midwifery for a small number of people whose main contribution would be in research. This should mirror the clinician scientist posts that exist in medicine, where a clinician carries a caseload within the clinical area but spends most time in research.

Finally, many of the participants wished to emphasise the positives about nursing and midwifery in Ireland. Those with a nursing and midwifery background were particularly keen to emphasise what they saw as an exciting period in the development of the professions and an exciting time to be involved. Great emphasis was placed on the need for concerted action from within the professions in order to get things done. Many said that people at the most senior level within the professions needed to engage and provide leadership:

> Educator: We have a lot of work to do and we have a lot of hard thinking to do and if we do not do it, we will miss the boat and that is irresponsible for anyone in our kind of positions in terms of the future of the profession in the country.

Skill Mix

Interviewee comments on skill mix are summarised in Table 23. Almost all interviewees favoured the concept of boundary spanning as a factor in skill mix. Many interviewees referred to the need for nursing and midwifery to spend time reflecting on what its core functions should be. As the role expands, and as health care assistants take on more responsibilities, and clerical and administrative staff take on functions that nurses and midwives previously did, it is important and necessary for the professions to reflect on what its core is.

One service manager spoke about nurses and midwives returning to Ireland having worked, for example, in the United

Table 23: Research Issues: Skill Mix

Theme	Frequency of mention
As the scope of nursing and midwifery practice expands, nurses and midwives will require the skill to span the boundaries between professions	72
There is a need for a more structured approach to skill mix within the clinical setting and to ensure that professionals are freed up to concentrate on their core job rather than being caught up in a lot of administrative duties	34
There will be a need to train and utilise to the full healthcare assistants as part of the skill mix in the nursing and midwifery settings	20
It is important to monitor the overall ratio of nurses and midwives to patients in Ireland	11
There will continue to be significant retention and recruitment issues in nursing and midwifery in Ireland and a resultant need to rely on nurses from other countries (e.g. India, the Philippines)	18

States, and experiencing frustration at not being able to do things they had formerly taken for granted. This was also discussed in the context of nurse-led services within the community or in smaller hospitals where, for example, there was a low requirement for X-rays and it made sense for nurses to be trained and empowered to take them when necessary. Some cited the example of the emergency medical technicians, whose role had expanded in recent years to prescribing, giving injections and other elements of emergency care.

One of the directors of the NMPDUs spoke about their intention to conduct an audit of the expansion of practice in their area to take stock of the skills that nurses and midwives had developed as part of their expanded practice and to assess whether or not they were still competent in those areas.

Another interviewee, a policymaker, expressed the move in this direction as follows:

> There is a reach upwards and there is a letting go of tasks and functions and I think that is something that has high value in a quality-focused health service.

Many practical examples were given. One medical consultant with a background in obstetrics described how duties that were once the responsibility of the doctor were now being performed by the midwife:

> In other aspects of intrapartum care, historically midwives have been the main prime caregivers but they have often expressed an interest in the possibility of doing ventouse deliveries or possibly foetal blood sampling in labour... duties that in the past have been duties of the doctor.

This interviewee said that this was more a case of midwives seeking and developing more autonomy and being keen to take on these roles rather than a case of doctors looking to hand them over, adding that this was something that was likely to increase in the future, a view that was shared by others.

Expansion of practice and boundary spanning were also frequently mentioned in the context of the EWTD, which was expected to have an impact on the availability of medical personnel and create pressure for nurses and midwives to take on roles that traditionally were done by doctors. Many interviewees felt that this was not a good basis for role development. There was a need for a more strategic assessment of what the role of the nurse and midwife should be within the services, rather than looking for them to fill gaps left by others.

Some talked about the difficulties within the services in relation to role expansion. In a move to modernise the service by expanding the role of nurses and midwives, some resistance was being experienced from medical unions, some doctors were 'precious... protective... and defensive' about their territory, and some nurses were 'holding onto their territory as well, with the care assistants aspiring to move into some of their patch'. There was, said a service manager, 'a lot of protection of old boundaries and still a lot of the demarcation mentality around'.

As the professions progressed to more community-based, nurse- or midwife-led services, boundary spanning was seen as becoming more prominent and more significant and an important message for patients and clients of the services:

> Service manager: Boundary spanning: we have got to get to a stage where that stroke patient and the family of that stroke patient, should find that, among his multidisciplinary team, there is one person who, no matter what the problem is, will take responsibility.

The degree of specialisation that the professions wished to promote and whether there was a long-term role for the generalist midwife was mentioned in relation to midwifery, in a setting where there were already five or six CMSs in areas such as cancer, urodynamics, diabetes and others:

> Medical consultant: Whether midwives should go totally specialised, in that they only work on the labour ward and don't work on the post-natal and antenatal, or whether they fulfil all the duties of the mid-wives and rotate between the wards, is a question that has never been decided in the profession as to what is the best way to go.

Other medical consultants spoke about 'the totality of care', which is at the heart of nursing, and involved spending time in conversation with the patients about their home circumstances and significant personal relationships, and the danger that this would disappear because they were busy doing many other things in the clinical area. Said one: 'the human dimension of health care delivery and service to patients must encapsulate that totality and we are becoming very clinical and that would worry me a little bit'.

A number of interviewees commented on recruitment and retention within nursing and midwifery. Most made reference to our increased dependency on internationally recruited nurses and wondered about the sustainability of this as a strategy. Others spoke about the difficulties of retaining nurses and midwives in the clinical area due to inflexible work practices and an increase in the medical and legal climate (especially in obstetrics). They said that nurse and midwife leaders should make it attractive for nurses and midwives to stay in nursing and midwifery, especially the young, well-educated entrants who will become the leaders of the future. This would include, for example, facilitating access to development opportunities for nurses and midwives and proactively supporting more flexible work practices. One nurse educator said that she was 'absolutely horrified' when she discovered that some qualified nurses had to give up their jobs at the height of a retention crisis in order to complete the post-registration bachelor of nursing studies (BNS) degree:

> There are still some pockets of unbelievable resistance and ignorance and lack of willingness to support staff in the system.

Another mentioned the 'unbelievably archaic structures in place in the mental health services, and they are pervasive', referring to practices such as central rostering, prioritising annual leave requests by seniority and other outdated HR and management practices, particularly in the voluntary sector of the mental health services. None of these approaches were seen as being conducive towards retaining and motivating staff within the professions.

Pre-Registration Education

The *Report of the Commission on Nursing* recommended that pre-registration nurse and midwife education should be at degree level in future. The transition to undergraduate education programmes leading to registration was completed in 2002, and was inevitably an important topic for discussion. See Table 24.

Table 24: Research Issues: Pre-Registration Education

Theme	Frequency of mention
There is a need to evaluate the effectiveness of the pre-registration education for nurses and midwives	84

The vast majority of interviewees saw the move to a baccalaureate pre-registration education programme as very positive, with one service manager describing it as 'the biggest single change in nursing in the last fifty years'. The move was viewed as giving nursing and midwifery an equal footing with other professions, enhancing their knowledge and understanding and helping them to become more confident in asking questions and demanding standards within the system. Interviewees also commented that nurses and midwives emerging from a degree programme would have a different view of themselves than their predecessors and would have higher expectations of their role, its positioning within the system and their own professional identity.

On the negative side, interviewees spoke about the dangers of removing nurses more and more from the bedside. Medical consultant interviewees, in particular, were concerned at some aspects of these developments. One said that in the education of doctors there had been a trend towards more integration into the clinical area, with more of an emphasis on skills rather than academic knowledge and that this mirrored the former rather than the present nursing and midwifery education system:

> Medical consultant: Nursing has gone hugely in a single generation in the opposite direction and I don't think that's ultimately going to work out well.

The consultant referred to the 'unpicking of academic orientation in medical training' and an increased emphasis on being 'more integrated into the clinical area, [and having] more skills focus, like nursing was'. Another medical consultant spoke about the danger of producing a theoretical nurse and not a practical nurse, and questioned whether 'the new order had gone too academic and not retained the important part because ultimately nursing is very practical and it must be practical'.

Not all medical consultants supported this view. One saw it as a positive development that should lead to more nurse-led developments:

> Medical consultant: There is still a hankering for the good old days. But when you actually go back and look at them they were not that good. The concern is that some of the sort of caring ethos could be lost in the academic model. That is a reasonable concern but I do not see any evidence to justify it.

The consultant went on to speak about nurse specialists in areas like diabetes and cystic fibrosis who have made a huge impact on the quality and continuity of care that patients get. The consultant felt that nursing was seriously under-utilised and said that the move of nursing towards more university-based education, pre- and post-registration, should contribute to a more sophisticated range of nurse-led roles.

Interviewees made some comments about the shape of the degree programme. Some felt that there should be a common point of entry to all branches of the professions. This would reflect what was happening in the UK and most other countries with a degree programme for nurse education. The common point of entry would entail all nurse and midwife students sharing a common first year or eighteen months at university and then choosing which branch they would take. The advantages of such a system would be the creation of greater interdisciplinary solidarity within the professions and the development of common standards across all the branches of the professions. As it stood, Ireland was the only country that had five separate undergraduate degree programmes (general, psychiatric, children's, and intellectual disability nursing, and midwifery).

One trade union representative, however, emphasised the advantages of developing individual degree programmes, with different points of entry, in order to ensure that the specific demands of each branch of the professions received sufficient attention. There was general agreement, however, that, while the five points of entry system was now well established in Ireland, it was likely to need review in the near future.

Some also suggested that the clinical year should be replaced with an internship, similar to that of medical students. Policymaker and educator interviewees said that, by 2010, the Bologna Declaration would take effect and this would involve a change to a three-year degree programme, followed by a year of internship. Many would agree with the comment from one service manager that 'there could be more of an emphasis on clinical placements'. A number of interviewees suggested that it was time now to conduct an evaluation of the degree programme, to review what changes needed to be made and what lessons had been learned. This would present the opportunity to examine again options such as single point of entry to nursing and midwifery, shared common basic education for nurse and midwife students, and the advisability or otherwise of sharing some education with other university-based students in areas such as science, medicine and other health disciplines.

Many interviewees believed that the changes in education for nurses and midwives would have a lasting and fundamental impact on the quality of nursing and midwifery. It was generally recognised that these changes were among the most important legacies of the Commission on Nursing:

> Educator: The impact of the Commission on Nursing has been huge and I don't think we will really be able to see the full impact for quite a while. The Commission on Nursing has lifted nursing out of a system of training that belonged to the beginning of the last century and it located nursing within the higher education sector. I think people will look back and will see it as having the equivalent impact to when nurses were first registered.

Post-Registration Education

Post-registration education is one way in which the broader issue of CPD is addressed, by providing the vehicle for the provision of formal educational programmes at postgraduate higher diploma and master levels. CPD, on the other hand, refers to the broader challenge that every professional faces of engaging in a lifelong process of continual refreshment of his or her knowledge and skills. Post-registration education is an important element of that. On post-registration education, Table 25 gives the principal topic of comment.

Table 25: Research Issues: Post-Registration Education

Theme	Frequency of mention
There is a need to evaluate the effectiveness of the post-registration education for nurses and midwives	91

Interviewees spoke about the need to ensure that post-registration education matched the needs of the service and of practice, and there was agreement that much progress had already been made: 'right around the country, we have tried to create programmes, both the service people and the university and educational people, to match the needs. I do think we have done a good job'.

An interviewee from one of the institutes of technology mentioned the importance of partnership relationships between the major providers of educational services in developing regionally based centres of expertise, rather than individual colleges looking to provide everything in each college. The big difference between the universities and the institutes of technology was that the latter were regionally based and focused on the needs of the region.

Interviewees said that that there was a need to differentiate between needs analysis at local and national levels. An NMPDU director spoke about the importance of doing proper needs analysis at unit level and developing local strategies that complemented national strategies, and referred to an initiative in their area where 'proper needs analysis tools are being developed regionally and are being given to all local managers'.

A number mentioned the discipline of conducting needs analysis on a regular basis, updating it in line with changing and evolving agendas, and, according to one service manager, 'matching to needs is something that would have to be kept very closely under review… on an ongoing basis'. An educator saw the need for a proactive rather than a reactive approach: a reactive approach seeks to 'address immediate situations' whereas what is required is a 'a more proactive approach, long term… what has been absent is the visionary ten- or twenty-year plan of where nurses will be, what will they be doing, who will be their client population'.

Another educator referred to the ongoing assessment of relevance to need:

> We need to remember that the agenda is evolving and, therefore, we need to be able to look honestly at our provision and drop parts of it when it is not appropriate and work in areas where it becomes necessary.

Some interviewees spoke about 'the shift in the community agenda', an emerging area of need that is not adequately addressed at present. There was a feeling that post-registration educational opportunities needed to be tailored to the emerging needs of professionals working in the community. As we have seen elsewhere in this research, there is an unstoppable shift in emphasis from acute settings to a population health model based on health education and promotion at community level and at providing services to patients in their own settings in the community. Post-registration educational opportunities needed to reflect this shift.

> NMPDU Director: Regarding population health, I think we need to reassess what we need to do within nurse education at undergraduate and postgraduate levels. We need to examine where we are going with education, now that we know what the new developments are going to be.

Another issue raised was access, accessibility and flexibility. An NMPDU director spoke about the need for postgraduate education programmes to be 'more accessible and flexible to nursing and midwifery students', in terms of 'greater variety of programmes… flexibility in entry requirements… in modular programmes' to suit the needs of the services and of nurses and midwives in a wide variety of service settings and personal circumstances.

Some said that programmes should demonstrate relevance to practice, and referred to the concept of 'learning contracts' and the importance of determining relevance to practice in the workplace in advance of study being undertaken and being approved. This kind of prior analysis of relevance could then be converted into a learning contract, under which the student contracted to achieve a level of skill and knowledge that was directly relevant to the needs of the unit at a local level. Allied to this was the impact on service:

> NMPDU director: One thing we are attempting to address now is having an impact on service, because sometimes you can run an awful lot of education and you are wondering if it is really impacting on the service.

A service manager was concerned about 'how relevant it is to corporate needs', stating that frequently education did not match those needs, quoting as an example 'training doctors to be more specialists, when what we want are more generalists... and we don't train them to work in teams'. A number of interviewees spoke about the importance of personal development planning from a personal, a professional and an organisational point of view.

Another service manager said it was important that education was not focused solely on the acquisition of knowledge but should also include the acquisition of relevant skills. A trade union representative termed this 'purposeful investment education and training... so that the people who come back with those skills are immediately put into a position where they can use them'.

The importance of protecting training budgets was mentioned by a service manager: 'education is as critical as trying to provide service needs but it has tended in the past to be one of the areas that suffers once there are cutbacks. Managers and nurse managers have to try to protect these resources'.

A number mentioned the establishment by the HSE of a post-registration nursing and midwifery education review group (PRERG).[249] This group is charged with the preparation of a comprehensive strategy for the development, delivery and evaluation of future post-registration nursing and midwifery education.

Continuing Professional Development

Two issues were discussed under the heading of CPD. Table 26 shows that most comments related to the need to evaluate the effectiveness of the provision of CPD for nurses and midwives. All interviewees endorsed the importance and value of CPD. Many stated that it should be a requirement of professionals to refresh their skills and knowledge periodically and this was best done through a modular system of CPD.

Table 26: Research Issues: Continuing Professional Development

Theme	Frequency of mention
There is a need to evaluate the effectiveness or otherwise of CPD as a way of addressing skills deficiencies in nurses and midwives	65
There is a need for greater use of opportunities to make joint clinical/educational appointments	5

Among the practical difficulties mentioned in association with CPD were access at a local level and staff release. The combination of difficulties in obtaining release for staff to attend courses, and the need for staff to travel distances to attend, militated against regular attendance by staff members who were very busy. Some commented that the failure to address these issues resulted in the wrong people attending CPD. This was summed up by a policymaker: 'people in the middle of their careers who are contributing the most are the ones who are participating the least'.

A number also said that CPD opportunities should reflect the circumstances of those who needed it. Another policymaker remarked:

> With predominantly female, higher numbers of flexible working, higher numbers of job-sharing, people not available for fulltime education as they are in fulltime employment… we have to have a more flexible, friendly approach to how we deliver educational packages.

Some spoke about getting staff released. An NMPDU director said, 'we are having huge difficulties getting staff released to undertake training'. This called for 'much more localised-based training within the sites, with e-learning and probably distance learning programmes for people to avail of education without necessarily impacting negatively on the service in terms of staff release'.

> Service manager: If you are going to be competent, you are going to have to provide evidence that you are attending courses that are appropriate.

This was seen as an important part of building a culture of personal professional accountability:

> Director of NMPDU: I see it as part of a cycle, once people are clear of their own accountability and what they need to keep up to speed with.

The interviewee went on to link this with the role that clinical audits could fulfil: 'if you have clinical audit or continuous quality initiatives, that will inform teams, including nurses, as to what skills people need, but that is an area that needs to be developed'. There was a link, therefore, between professional accountability, quality and clinical audits, and an important potential role for clinical audits at a team level that considered the skill mix within the overall team.

Interviewees mentioned the lack of proper evaluation of those programmes that were on offer and the lack of an overall analysis of the CPD needs of the profession that could form the basis for the development of a coordinated strategy. This made it difficult to assess whether those courses offered value for money or had an impact on the skill levels of those who attended. The provision of CPD should be in line with what was needed:

> Service manager: There has to be a regular sampling of programmes that the taxpayer is paying for to see if that is what is required.

Some linked the development of a coordinated strategy for CPD to the wider question of professional development, performance appraisal and review. It should be, they said, an integral part of the HR systems that existed within the profession that people were given proper feedback on their performance through an appraisal system and an opportunity to discuss a development programme that met their own professional needs and the needs of the service within which they worked. An educator and an NMPDU director both commented that such a system would also contribute towards the development of more practice-relevant CPD opportunities, as the nature of the needs of the professionals and of the service would become clearer and feed into the development of educational interventions.

A number of interviewees specifically mentioned the publication by the National Council of the *Guidelines for Portfolio Development for Nurses and Midwives*.[250] Portfolio development was seen as a useful tool in the wider education and development of the individual, as it provided a stimulus to examine wider educational opportunities and needs. It was also seen as a practical way of integrating professional development into the clinical area and taking account of experience.

A number of interviewees commented on the opportunities presented by CPD for interdisciplinary and multidisciplinary educational opportunities:

> Trade Union: Multidisciplinary, now that is where CPD comes in – and it should be more multidisciplinary.... We have to talk to one another, everyone being in their own silos. It is still there and we have not done a great deal to break down those walls.

The directors of CNEs/CMEs commented on the disappointment they felt about the lack of integration between the clinical and third-level setting. A typical comment was:

> CNE director: In some instances, a lot of people coordinating the undergraduate programmes at the universities never had any experience in the area. In fact quite the opposite, and with regard to the lack of integration between the university and the clinical setting, we were told there would be shared learning and lecture-practitioners. The university people rarely visit the clinical setting and, if they do, it is a social visit and that is poor integration of theory and practice.

Medical consultants, in particular, commented on what they saw as the consolidation of a divide between the clinical setting and the academic setting by the lack of involvement of senior lecturers and professors of nursing in clinical settings. They said that, despite the many criticisms that were made of 'the medical model', it was one aspect that the profession of medicine valued very highly. With the exception of basic education at the very beginning of their careers, medical students were taught by practising clinicians. The professions had resisted attempts to shift towards the academic paradigm of pure research and pure teaching, because of what they perceived as the immense value of maintaining those close links between academia, clinical practice and research. There was 'no reason why there should not be lecturers, senior lecturers and professors of nursing working on the wards'.

Common Education

The topic of common education generated considerable comment, which is reviewed in Table 27 under seven main headings. Almost all interviewees saw only advantages in common education.

Table 27: Research Issues: Common Education

Theme	Frequency of mention
There are advantages associated with the development of common education opportunities for clinical professionals from different disciplines	121
There are disadvantages associated with the development of common educational opportunities for clinical professionals from different disciplines	4
Common training in communication skills should be included as part of a common education curriculum	34
Training in financial skills should be included as part of a common education curriculum	5
A general introduction to health economics should be included as part of a common education curriculum	2
Training in management and administration systems should be included as part of a common education curriculum	20
A common education curriculum should include training in teamworking skills	22

One policymaker spoke about the value of 'common basic education for clinical professionals', while one director of an NMPDU commented:

> When we educate all disciplines together we will break down these silos and each see how the other profession fits in.

Some interviewees said that, in addition to developing shared educational opportunities in some areas of the clinical curriculum, students should also be offered common courses in areas such as communications, teamworking and management. As one medical consultant put it:

> If we are going to be working as a team, then we should be training as a team.

The advantages of such a system include the creation of opportunities for clinical professionals to understand each other better and the contribution that their discipline makes to the health services. It would create the opportunity for improved communication between the disciplines, building greater mutual respect and fostering a spirit of teamwork as a basis for enhanced multidisciplinary cooperation in the clinical setting.

> CNE director: Common education will help. You see very diverse professionals there and if they can actually manage to get together, then there certainly is hope for the future with regards to teamworking.

Many interviewees suggested that this approach would introduce a radical transformation of the culture of the professions. In nursing and midwifery, one service manager described the hierarchy of the branches as 'general nursing is number one, psychiatry falls in at number two and then there is midwifery and the rest'.

The same, it was said, was true of the relations between the professions, where a definite hierarchy existed. Learning and working together in college would help to eradicate this mentality and generate a greater respect for the respective roles of each of the professions and the branches within the professions.

Within the educational system, there were moves in this direction. A number of interviewees mentioned a pilot project for a higher diploma in neonatal intensive care, using funding provided by the National Council. The course was multidisciplinary in nature and was being delivered to mixed groups of nurses, midwives and doctors.

A service manager observed that the development of common education opportunities was seen as likely to lead to an increase in the modular approach to course design, with an increase in interchange between disciplines and between colleges. This was in line with the spirit of the Bologna Declaration, referred to earlier, where interchange between colleges and courses would increase opportunities for students to build their competence and education around targeted needs and their own strengths.

Conclusions

Based on the research in this and earlier chapters, the key professional development implications for the future role of nursing and midwifery in Ireland, as perceived by the stakeholders who took part in this research, can be summarised as follows:

- A single point of entry to the professions of nursing and midwifery should be provided, based on a common initial year in which the core elements of nursing and midwifery practice are emphasised. Subsequent division into specialised areas of practice should also include as much as possible elements of integrated, interdisciplinary education. This is an important element in developing and promoting a strong professional identity within the professions. This recommendation also anticipates the implications of the Bologna Declaration.

- A comprehensive and rich career pathway for nurses and midwives in clinical, management, education, research and professional development should exist, supported by the provision of a comprehensive range of educational, training and development opportunities at pre-registration and post-registration levels.
- Joint appointments, in line with agreed frameworks and protocols, should be encouraged and available across all the career pathways.
- A detailed description of the competencies required for each career pathway in nursing and midwifery should be provided.
- The role of nurses and midwives should be developed in accordance with agreed frameworks for the expansion of practice, practice development, accreditation of education and training provision, approval of posts, registration requirements and professional development provisions.
- The development of the role of nurses and midwives, including the determination of the numbers that will be required within each pathway and at each level of practice/ management grade, should be determined based on a strategic assessment of service needs.
- The direct entry degree programmes should include some elements of common basic education, through the development of modules within the degree programmes that are common.
- Direct entry degree programmes should explore possibilities for multidisciplinary educational opportunities where this is feasible, through the development of modules targeted at health care professionals from other disciplines.
- Opportunities should continue to be developed for access to registration in the other branches of the professions for registered nurses and midwives, through post-registration education programmes.
- A comprehensive professional career development service should be provided for all nurses and midwives.
- Continuing professional development should be incorporated into HR management practices, including a comprehensive

system of performance appraisal, personal development plans and peer review.

- In recruitment practices, particular attention should be given to the possibility of joint appointments across the various career pathways. The potential for joint appointments should be explored and promoted wherever possible.
- HR managers should work with nurse and midwife managers in all career pathways to increase the attractiveness of the professions for potential entrants.
- Registered nurses and midwives should be required to produce evidence of professional development activities in line with guidelines to be agreed. These guidelines would include a description of the responsibilities of individual nurses and midwives and of managers in this area.
- A comprehensive institutional framework should continue to exist and to be developed for the provision of post-registration education and training.
- National and regional support agencies should continue to exist, with responsibility for the strategic planning and development of the professions in line with the needs of the services and the evolving role of nurses and midwives within the services.
- Universal access to professional development opportunities should be a key principle in the development of programmes.
- Post-registration educational and training provision should continue to be developed in a manner that reflects the evolving needs of the service and the professions and, in particular, the career pathways within the professions.
- The development and provision of professional development post-registration opportunities should be undertaken with an emphasis on supporting nurses and midwives in the expansion of their practice in line with the framework for scope of practice and the needs of the services.
- Particular attention should be paid to the development of professional development opportunities in the area of primary care where a lack of provision has been identified.
- Post-registration educational opportunities should develop where appropriate on a multidisciplinary basis, integrating education for nurses and midwives in specialist areas with the provision of education for other health care professionals.

- Nurses and midwives in all career pathways and at all levels of practice should be encouraged and supported in developing succession planning and fast-tracking initiatives aimed at enhancing the competence profile of nurses and midwives in all areas and ensuring that an adequate supply of competent professionals exists capable of filling roles and posts as they become available in line with the needs of the services and of patients and clients.
- Professional development opportunities should be made available for the development of management and leadership competencies in all career pathways.
- Opportunities should be made available for the development of expertise in the use and integration of ICT into the delivery of health care services by nurses and midwives.
- Nurses and midwives should be provided with regular information and educational opportunities that build an understanding of the health care services, the public sector, standards of public accountability, governance, risk management and health economics, public–private partnerships and other themes that enhance their understanding of the context within which services are provided.
- Continuing professional development should include education and training on cultural issues in the delivery of services, including an appreciation of the multi-ethnic nature of Irish society and the importance of sensitivity and understanding of cultural differences.
- Nurses and midwives should be provided with access to post-registration training and educational opportunities on a multidisciplinary basis in areas that enhance their ability to make a contribution to the efficiency and effectiveness of the services.
- Programmes in interprofessional education should be encouraged with a renewed emphasis on building into these programmes an evaluation of their effectiveness.
- Local and regional providers of services in the area of post-registration professional development should collaborate with users of these services to assess local need and effectiveness.
- A comprehensive professional development strategy should include the creation of opportunities to prepare nurses and

midwives to deliver meaningful inputs into the strategic planning of the executive functions of the health services, health care policy and performance management and monitoring arrangements. This will be aimed at ensuring that the professions of nursing and midwifery are capable of providing both the Department of Health and Children and the HSE with competent professionals capable of having a meaningful input at the highest levels.

Part 3

The Strategic Challenges

Chapter 11

Strategic Issues for Nursing and Midwifery in Ireland

The aim of this chapter is to provide the basis for a strategy for the professional development of nursing and midwifery for the ten-year period 2008–2017. The strategy is not intended as a static plan but as a dynamic planning and development instrument that should evolve and develop to meet changes in the environment. The choice of a ten-year period within which to frame the strategy is a pragmatic one. It is based on good practice in business and organisational strategic planning, areas that require the setting of realistic timescales within which the effectiveness of a strategy can be measured. It is also predicated on the basis of a rolling review each year, with substantial reviews in years 5 and 9.

The choice of a ten-year timescale for the strategy is apt at the present time because 2008 marks the tenth anniversary of the publication of the *Report of the Commission on Nursing*, which has provided a reference point by which to measure progress and changes made in nursing and midwifery in Ireland. Almost all the recommendations of the Commission on Nursing have been implemented. One notable exception is the passing of a new Nurses Act to replace the *Nurses Act, 1985* but, at the time of writing, plans are well underway to address this deficit. The legacy of the Commission on Nursing is there to be seen. This proposed strategy is intended to answer the following questions: what is the next step? And what will nursing and midwifery feel and look like ten years from now?

The structure of the strategy, as outlined in this chapter, is based on the experience of strategic planning that has been accumulated in the National Council from 2001 to date. It follows standard business planning templates but is adapted to the specific circumstances of nursing and midwifery. The elements of the strategy can be summarised as follows:

- **Analysis**: A summary of the strengths, weaknesses, opportunities and threats (SWOT) facing the professions of nursing and midwifery in Ireland today; this is an essential preamble to the development of strategies to take advantage of the strengths, resolve the weaknesses, exploit the opportunities and avoid the threats.
- **Vision**: This will state what nursing and midwifery should look and feel like in the health services of the future, and in particular in ten years time, at the end of the period of this strategy.
- **Mission statement**: This will address the question, what is the central role and purpose of nursing and midwifery in the health services?
- **Values**: This suggests what the core values of the professions of nursing and midwifery should be, based on an understanding of the essence of nursing and midwifery and their mission within the services.
- **Objectives**: This will state what the long-term objectives of the strategy should be, in line with the expectations and requirements of all the major stakeholders. These objectives should reflect the underlying reasons for being involved in the delivery of professional nursing and midwifery services and should be related to the outputs and the outcomes that nurses and midwives seek to deliver.
- **Key strategies**: These are the rules and guidelines by which the mission and objectives may be achieved. These will be based on the SWOT analysis and will seek to build on the strengths, resolve the weaknesses, exploit the opportunities and avoid the threats.
- **Strategic action programmes**: This is an action plan, outlined in Chapter 12, that sets out how the key strategies will be implemented. It will cover issues such as objectives, resources, timescales, deadlines and performance indicators.
- **Conclusion and next steps**: Chapter 12 provides a brief outline of the next steps involved in generating ownership of the strategy at a national level and the importance of the negotiation and development process that will be required to implement it.

SWOT Analysis

Based on the outcomes of the research, including the comments made by interviewees and participants in focus groups, Table 28 is a summary of the principal strengths, weaknesses, opportunities and threats that are relevant for the development of a strategy for the professional development of nursing and midwifery.

Table 28: SWOT Analysis of Nursing and Midwifery in Ireland

Strengths	**Weaknesses**
• Structures and policies • Professional development • Education • Clinical credibility • Workforce	• Leadership • Skill mix • Integration • Service development • Capacity in the community
Opportunities	**Threats**
• Structures and policies • Professional development • Education • Legislation • Workforce	• Identity • Professional development capacity • Recruitment and retention • Capacity in the community • Clinical involvement

Strengths

The research points to many significant strengths in nursing and midwifery in Ireland today. They can be summarised under the headings shown in Table 28 (top left-hand box):

Structures and Policies

The existence of a single structure for the management and delivery of health care in Ireland was seen as a very positive development by participants in this research, notwithstanding the criticisms of some aspects of the delivery system and the way in which it was introduced. Overall, the Health Service Reform Programme and the reports and policy documents that underpin it were welcomed as a significant step forward. For nursing and midwifery, a particular strength over the last ten years was the implementation of the recommendations of the *Report of the Commission on Nursing*. This has been instrumental in revolutionising nursing and midwifery in Ireland, not least by the provision of a clearly defined clinical career pathway, the role of the National Council, the creation of institutional frameworks for the development of the professions, the creation of the nursing policy unit within the Department of Health and Children and the reform and investment in education and professional development. While not mentioned specifically by the Commission on Nursing, the creation of HIQA was also welcomed as an important dimension in the accountability structures for the services.

Professional Development

The profile and provision of professional development for nursing and midwifery emerged from this research as a great strength; in particular, the structures and frameworks that are in place and the expertise that has been built up in the National Council and in the NMPDUs. This has resulted in clinical career pathways being clearly defined and implemented. This progress has been complemented by the creation of a portfolio approach to career planning. Recent work in professional development has built on the *Scope of Nursing and Midwifery Practice Framework* that was put in place in 2000. This framework has provided the professions with a solid platform upon which to expand their practice while still retaining their distinct identities. The research also highlighted evidence of expanding practice for nursing and midwifery. In addition to initiatives in the expansion of practice, there has been specialisation and advanced practice in nursing and midwifery and this is being implemented proactively throughout the service. Finally, the research also highlighted the important benefits from the introduction of legislation providing for the involvement of nurses and midwives in the prescription of medical preparations and the creation of the structures necessary to make this happen.

Education

The substantial investment in education for nurses and midwives in recent years was identified by this research as a major strength for the professions, particularly the introduction of the pre-registration degree programme for all the branches of the professions and the development of enriched post-registration education opportunities. The research also pointed to the value of work that is currently underway in the area of post-registration education. In addition to the formal education structures, a wide range of opportunities for CPD are now in place. The centres for nurse education were seen as being of great importance in the provision of important skills development and training.

Clinical Credibility
The research showed the continued credibility that the professions of nursing and midwifery enjoy within the health services in Ireland. This is evidenced by the good working relationships that exist between nursing and midwifery and medical consultants and the predominantly positive image of the professions that is held by many service managers. The expansion of nursing and midwifery practice, the development of specialists and advanced practice and the increase in the number and variety of nurse-/midwife-led services in acute and primary settings are all reasons why the professions enjoy an enhanced reputation and credibility with the health services. This is a strength that was pervasive throughout all of the research, notwithstanding the weaknesses and threats that were also identified.

Workforce
In addition to having achieved a considerable degree of respect and credibility as clinical professions, nurses and midwives are also seen as a committed, flexible and adaptive workforce. This came through in many instances within the research, despite some of the difficulties that were also identified. On the whole, the professions are regarded as being populated by a caring, committed workforce.

Weaknesses
The research also identified important weaknesses for the professions, which are summarised under the headings shown in Table 28 (top right-hand box).

Leadership
Ten years on, the research undertaken for this book broadly replicates the findings of the Commission on Nursing pertaining to the lack of strong leadership in nursing and midwifery in Ireland. The effects of this lack of leadership manifest themselves in many ways but perhaps most importantly in an absence of

communication, coordination and integration in nursing and midwifery across the divisions of the Register, institutional settings and grades. As a result, there is a lack of professional identity and of clear direction in nursing and midwifery and a deficiency of voice and credibility at the decision-making table. The research also highlighted a continued negative, destructive culture of bullying and divisiveness. There continues to be a low level of participation in, and availability of, CPD opportunities for staff nurses and midwives, despite the significant increase in provision. The absence of professional identity and leadership also manifests itself in a lack of research capacity and competence within the professions, although progress is being made though the implementation of the Department of Health and Children´s nursing and midwifery research strategy. The research in this book indicates a slow uptake of opportunities for joint appointments, and it will require strong leadership across the academic/clinical divide to improve this. The negative influence of trade unions within the professions was mentioned in the research, reflected in the promotion of resistance to change, creating bitter divisions between nursing and midwifery management and staff and undermining the role of the director of nursing and midwifery. Finally, while the research welcomed the post of chief nursing officer with a team of nursing advisors within the Department, their role and function remained unclear and undefined in the context of the Health Service Reform Programme. The impact of this role has yet to be felt.

Skill Mix

This is an unresolved issue in nursing and midwifery. The research emphasised the importance of skill mix in the recruitment and retention of nurses and midwives. Experience from the United Kingdom, United States and Canada points to the importance of creating attractive working environments that act as magnets to staff to work. This requires investment in skill at all levels and across all grades and the development of complementarity within and between roles. The question of skill mix is particularly important in the development of multidisciplinary teams in acute and primary care settings. Recent demands for the introduction of a thirty-five hour week for nurses and midwives and the creation of a commission to review the thirty-five hour week have raised the importance of the need for skill mix developments.

Integration

This is a key theme for the health services for the future. The research noted that one of the weaknesses of the new HSE organisational structures was the creation of separate pillars for primary care (PCCC) and acute care (NHO). This only serves to emphasise lack of integration within the structures of the HSE itself and makes it difficult to achieve the objectives of the transformation programme, which has at its centre the concept of a shift towards community-based services and the creation of an acute–primary care continuum (see HSE update, page 61). The research also suggested that there was a lack of integration across the professions, as has been already mentioned as part of the weakness in leadership. Finally, the research also pointed to the confusion that exists about the nature of the changes in the role of the Department of Health and Children, which does not serve well the need for an integrated approach to planning and delivery.

Service Development

The research emphasised the importance of service development as an important part of the changes in organisational structures in the future. In particular, it emphasised the need to put the patient/client at the centre of service development. The research further emphasised the need for an integrated service development framework for nurse- and midwife-led services and the provision of support and training in service development for nurses and midwives. This is an essential corollary to the rollout of the HSE's transformation programme.

Capacity in the Community

One of the national goals of the health services is to ensure the system has the capacity to deliver timely and effective health care services. However, the research revealed concerns about capacity problems creating pressures within the system. Given the emphasis on integration of services and the shift to the community, concerns have been raised about nursing and midwifery capacity within the community. In the area of mental health services, the *Vision for Change*[151] report noted that there were not enough psychiatric nurses in the community to meet the needs arising from a continued shift of services away from institutional settings and said that there was a need to build up community mental health teams, which will require the creation of multidisciplinary community-based capacity. The transformation programme emphasises the importance of the primary care teams (PCTs). If these are to function correctly, they will also require capacity building in the community. A mapping exercise conducted by the HSE estimated that 500 PCTs would be required and that the minimum core team members would include GPs, practice nurses, occupational therapists, PHNs, physiotherapists, speech and language therapists, social workers and home helps. Also included in this team should be general nurses and midwives, nurse and midwife specialists and advanced nurse and advanced midwife practitioners and other support workers. The intention is that social care networks would link these teams. A total of 130 such networks would be required, linking three-to-five people teams for population bases of 30,000 to 50,000 people. Nurses and midwives are important elements of PCTs and building capacity to meet this need is a major challenge. The research recognised that, in order to meet capacity requirements, it is likely that there will be a need to increase the capacity of private sector provision.

Opportunities

The research highlighted opportunities for the professions of nursing and midwifery in the future. These are summarised under the headings shown in Table 28 (bottom left-hand box):

Structures and Policies

The HSE´s transformation programme presents nursing and midwifery with the potential to make a major impact on shaping the health services of the future. It provides an ideal opportunity for creating innovative nurse- and midwife-led services and plays a central role in setting up and ensuring the effectiveness of the PCTs. The nursing policy division in the Department of Health and Children and the nursing unit in the HSE also provide nursing and midwifery with the potential to access policy formulation and service planning at the highest level. The introduction of prescribing for nurses and midwives is an opportunity for the professions to add an important new dimension to their practice in a way that meets the needs of patients and clients. The commission set up to review the possibility of introducing a thirty-five hour week offers scope for nurses and midwives to look at their work practices and the skill-mix issues in their work settings and provide innovative solutions to achieving a thirty-five hour week without significant additions to cost in terms of whole time equivalents. The emergence of active representative patient and consumer groups is an opportunity for nurses and midwives to engage with them in a manner that emphasises the patient-centred nature of nursing and midwifery care. The National Treatment Purchase Fund and other public–private partnership initiatives within the services enable nursing and midwifery to ensure that professional development extends beyond the public sector to encompass all of the professions, regardless of work settings.

Professional Development

The research underscored the progress that has been made to date on a wide range of professional development opportunities for the professions and also drew attention to the importance of the role of the National Council. The National Council was set up to promote the role of nursing and midwifery in line with service need in public, voluntary and private settings and this emphasis on service need has been a hallmark of its work. The continuance of this work presents opportunities to continue to provide leadership in the development of nursing and midwifery in a manner that is responsive to the needs of the service and of patients and clients. The research also emphasised the importance of the emergence of integrated care pathways as a basis for both professional and service development. Another opportunity for the professions is the emerging increased volume of multidisciplinary cooperation in service and in education. The research noted the value of joint appointments as opportunities for the professions to build a strong sense of professional identity and a strong culture of academic and evidence-based clinical practice, which is enhanced by the evidence of increasing integration of university and hospital networks. Finally, the research called attention to the opportunities resulting from the ongoing implementation of the Department of Health and Children´s research strategy.

Education

Earlier chapters have outlined the many opportunities for nursing and midwifery as a result of the major investment in education for nurses and midwives over the past ten years. The increased education activity in universities and institutes of technology and in the centres for nurse education offers a rich vein of potential for the profession, not least of all in the development of academic competence and research capacity. The combination of the emphasis on multidisciplinary education at undergraduate and postgraduate levels and the increasing volume of post-registration education signals the potential for a wide range of opportunities, hitherto unimagined by many nurses and midwives.

Legislation

The Government is expected to introduce a new Nurses and Midwives Act in the near future. This is an opportunity for the regulation and development of the professions in a manner that capitalises on the strengths of the progress that has been made since the publication of the *Report of the Commission on Nursing*. International best practice in this area indicates the need for enabling and flexible legislation that creates the conditions for the professions to develop in a manner that is responsive to the needs of the service and of patients and clients. One of the principal aims of the legislation will be to protect the public through strong regulatory structures and processes. It is important, however, that the legislation should also distinguish between this function (which is the remit of the regulatory body) and the proactive development of the professions (which is the remit of the services). Legislation should not hamper the ability of the professions to develop in line with the needs of the service.

Workforce

Nursing and midwifery in Ireland enjoys a very good reputation and the workforce is highly regarded. The evidence presented in earlier chapters has shown that there is a great deal of goodwill within the professions and willingness to adapt to meet the challenges of the future, a fact that leaders of the professions must seize upon.

Threats

A number of potential threats have already been identified that could undermine the potential of the professions to fulfil their destiny within the health services of the future (see Table 28, bottom right-hand box).

Identity

One of the biggest threats is the potential for a loss of professional identity in the health services of the future. Nursing and midwifery must remain true to itself as it evolves along the clinical career pathway and develops nurse-/midwife-led services. This raises the importance of nursing and midwifery maintaining contact with the essence of nursing. Another significant factor is the lack of cohesiveness within nursing and midwifery. This can occur because of a lack of leadership and empowerment or as a result of poorly managed industrial unrest. Ten years ago the Commission on Nursing noted that the professions could be destructive, negative and litigious, adjectives that can still be applied today. The research commented on the negative impact of trade unions that have promoted an industrial relations culture that is detrimental to the professional identity of nurses and midwives. The lack of professional identity was frequently alluded to and manifested by the continuing disempowerment of nurses and midwives within the services. These two factors represent a threat to the professions´ ability to perceive themselves as an empowered workforce, confident and clear about their key role as central players in the development and delivery of the services of the future. This threat, now identified, must be confronted.

Professional Development Capacity

The *Prospectus Report* recommended that the functions of the National Council should be divided between and transferred to the HSE and An Bord Altranais. In effect this would amount to dissolution of the National Council and a division of its activities between the two organisations. The National Council´s capacity for leading on professional development and its many achievements has been widely acknowledged by individual nurses and midwives and service providers alike. Examples of its leadership activities include encouraging the professions to adapt to role change, facilitating the development of roles within frameworks for practice, promoting the integration of services, developing new skills that are required, building opportunities for and participation in CPD, and promoting opportunities for interdisciplinary education. All these activities have been undertaken with the needs of patients, clients and the services in mind. The loss of the National Council thus poses a real threat to nursing and midwifery in public, voluntary and private care settings, in that the expertise in professional development could be lost to the professions. It would also be a threat to the development of appropriate services in line with the evolving needs of the service, of patients and clients.

Recruitment and Retention

The professions face threats arising from difficulties in recruiting and retaining staff both at present and in the future. The literature reviewed has confirmed that this is not just a threat in Ireland. The challenge now is for policymakers, service planners and service managers to ensure that the capacity exists to meet the service needs of the future by recruiting and retaining a cohort of competent and motivated nursing and midwife professionals.

Capacity in the Community

The lack of community-based capacity within the professions is a significant threat, given the central importance of building community-based services, encouraging a shift away from acute services and developing a service continuum between acute and primary care.

Clinical Involvement

As reform of the health service progresses, it is important that decision-making in relation to health care is not driven solely by considerations of economic efficiency. This can result in cuts and changes being made that are not in the best interests of patients and clients and of the services. As service managers come under increased pressure to deliver services constrained by tight budgets and with full accountability for those services, there is a danger that services will be closed or reduced without due consideration of the outcomes of these closures and reductions. It is essential that clinical involvement in decision-making about resource allocation is further refined and extended at national, regional and local levels. This also includes decision-making about the structures and processes that will be in place within the services of the future for the professional development of nursing and midwifery. As organisational change and structural reform roll out, pressure has built up for the forthcoming Nurses and Midwives Act to define the role of regulation, the fundamental concern of which is the protection of the public rather than professional development. Regulation by its nature is legalistic and works in a culture that is very different from the developmental, innovative culture of professional development. While of paramount importance, the regulatory role should not impede professional development and careful consideration needs to be given to the involvement of the clinical expertise that has been built up over the past ten years in the development of the professions.

Responding to SWOT Analysis

This concludes the SWOT analysis of the professions of nursing and midwifery based on the literature review and the results of the research presented in earlier chapters. These considerations provide the material for appropriate responses in the form of strategies and action plans to build on the strengths, tackle the weaknesses, exploit the opportunities and avoid the threats. Looking into the future of the health services from the perspective gained through this SWOT analysis, it is time now to consider what nursing and midwifery should be like in ten years´ time as a result of implementing a strategic development plan.

A Vision of Nursing and Midwifery

What should nursing and midwifery in Ireland look and feel like in ten years time? What will it be like to be a nurse and midwife in Ireland at that time? Informed by the findings of this research, the principal dimensions of the vision for nursing and midwifery in the health services in Ireland by the year 2017 are professional identity, opportunities for ongoing education and professional development, strong leadership and visibility as leaders in all health care settings, and greater cohesion and integration within the professions across settings and sectors. What follows are vision statements relating to these principal dimensions:

- The professions of nursing and midwifery will enjoy a strong professional identity. Nurse and midwife leaders will be prominent in the formulation of policy for the health services and in the development of service plans to implement that policy. Communication and coordination within the professions will create the platform for the generation of credible public positions that will articulate their contribution to the health services and act as an advocate on behalf of patients and clients of the service. Nursing and midwifery will continue to be seen as a desirable career option and will have a reputation for retaining staff.
- Nurses and midwives will enjoy access to rich and rewarding educational and professional development opportunities adapted to their area of practice. These will be predominantly interdisciplinary in nature, involving interaction with other professions and support workers.
- Nurses and midwives will work either as leaders or members of care teams in every health care setting. This will involve an identification of the specific contribution that each member of the team makes to the achievement of the goals of the service. Increasingly, these teams will involve a wider mix of skills aimed at ensuring that each of the members of the team maximises their specific contribution.
- Nurses and midwives will be highly visible within the community as leaders of nursing and midwifery services and as members of primary care teams involving other professionals and support services, including nurse- and midwife-led clinics and home-based services. This will include nurses and midwives at every stage of the clinical career pathway, from generalist to specialist to advanced practice.
- Nurses and midwives, at generalist, specialist and advanced practice levels, will complement and augment the work of GPs in the delivery of patient-centred services, frequently within the patient´s own home and family setting. The nurse

and midwife will be a resource to families and communities in addressing all their health needs, including referring individuals on to other professional services in primary and acute settings. Nurses and midwives will be the main coordinators of care in the community.

- Nurses and midwives will occupy a central role in the education of individuals, their families and the community in the promotion of good health. This will be seen to deliver measurable outcomes in areas such as lifestyle diseases. This will complement the emergence of more informed patients and clients, interested in being involved in managing their own health and well-being.
- Nurses and midwives will continue to occupy a central role in the development of acute hospital services, including generalist, specialist and advanced practice in a manner that ensures that the patient remains at the centre of acute care provision. The nurse and midwife will play a central role in coordinating the inputs of other health care professionals. The nurse and midwife will also ensure that continuity of care is provided across the acute/primary care divide by following up with the patients and clients in their own homes and coordinating with community-based care services to deliver follow-up care.
- There will be a significant increase in the use of joint appointments along the career pathway for nurses and midwives. They will be involved in research, education and clinical practice increasingly on the basis of shared contracts between different institutional settings.

Mission Statement

A mission statement in this context seeks to define the central role and purpose of nursing and midwifery in the future Irish health services. This definition is based largely on the needs of the service as identified in the research and the essence of nursing and is as follows:

Nurses and midwives in Ireland will provide a comprehensive range of care services to individuals and their families, across all institutional health care settings, in close cooperation with other health care professionals and support workers. The provision of this care will be inspired by the following considerations:

- **Person-centred**: Nursing and midwifery will provide person-centred care to individuals and their families based on an understanding of their specific needs. In doing this the nurse and midwife will act at all times in the interests of the person.
- **Relationship-based**: In the provision of patient-centred care, nurses and midwives will build up a relationship based on empathy with the individual, based on respect and consideration and animated by the values of equality, esteem, meaning, safety and trust.
- **Holistic**: The care provided by the nurse and midwife will focus on the totality of the person, physical, psychosocial and emotional. It will also be sensitive to the cultural circumstances of the individual and be based on the values of respect for diversity and equality.
- **Education and information**: The care provided by the nurse or midwife will focus on promoting self-reliance and independence in the individual. This will include providing them with the wherewithal to become independent. It will extend beyond the individual to their families and communities in order to ensure that support mechanisms are empowered to assist.
- **Coordination**: Nurses and midwives will ensure that the individual has access to whatever is required to assist them to achieve self-reliance and independence. This will include coordinating the inputs of other professionals, making technology available as required and taking charge of environmental management issues that affect their well-being.
- **Continuity**: Nurses and midwives will provide care in whatever setting best meets the needs of the individual and of the services. This will include acute and primary settings and will involve spanning the boundaries of both by following the patient throughout the system. In providing this care, the nurse and midwife will act as part of a multidisciplinary team, either as member or as leader, as needed.
- **Knowledge and skills**: Nurses and midwives will invest in their own education and development, fully aware that

clinical wisdom comes about as a result of experience combined with knowledge and understanding. Competence development will be seen as an essential ingredient in the accountability values that nurses and midwives build into their professional practice. Nurses and midwives will see themselves as professionals who combine science and art in the interests of the individual under their care. This will also include the acquisition of specialist knowledge aimed at providing an enhanced level of care to target groups.

Values

The values that govern the work and conduct of nurses and midwives in their professional lives are outlined in the *Code of Professional Conduct for each Nurse and Midwife.*[252] This provides nurses and midwives with a framework within which to make decisions and is also intended to promote high standards of professional conduct. The values contained in the code reflect the essence of nursing and are relevant in the context of this strategy. They can be summarised as follows:

- **Accountability**: Nurses and midwives are accountable for their own practice
- **Safety**: The safety of those in their care is of paramount importance
- **Confidentiality**: Nurses and midwives do not divulge information about those in their care
- **Trust**: Nurses and midwives do not betray the trust placed in them by patients and clients
- **Information**: Nurses and midwives provide patients with information on their care in an appropriate manner
- **Sexual propriety and respect**: Nurses and midwives do not make sexual advances to those in their care
- **Competence**: Nurses and midwives base their professional judgement on their competence, which they have a duty to maintain. They also acknowledge when appropriate the limits of their competence
- **Conscience/conscientiousness**: Nurses and midwives make known any conscientious objections they may have to practices

- **Shared responsibility**: Nurses and midwives share the responsibility for care with other colleagues and must ensure that workload pressures do not jeopardise that care
- **Education**: Nurses and midwives have a duty to educate junior staff and to ensure that responsibilities are not delegated beyond levels of competence
- **Responsibility and accountability**: Nurses and midwives are responsible and accountable for the care provided by students under their supervision
- **Cooperation**: Nurses and midwives cooperate with health care professionals and others to promote the health of the public
- **Life**: Nurses and midwives work to preserve human life and, when death is imminent, to ensure that the patient dies with dignity
- **Public statements**: Nurses and midwives make it clear when speaking in public whether they are expressing a personal or a professional opinion
- **Commerce/commercialisation**: Nurses and midwives do not use professional qualifications to promote commercial products
- **Gifts**: Nurses and midwives do not accept gifts or favours that could be interpreted as wishing to exert undue influence or obtain preferential treatment
- **Personal health**: Nurses and midwives take precautions to ensure that their state of health enables them to be competent in fulfilling their duties. Abuse of drugs and alcohol adversely affects that competence
- **Research ethics**: Nurses and midwives have a responsibility to adhere to high standards of ethical practice in conducting or participating in research.

Objectives

The long-term objectives of the professions of nursing and midwifery must be to meet the expectations and requirements of all the major stakeholders in the health services, i.e. individual patients and clients, the general public, professional colleagues and co-workers, employers, policymakers and the Government. The objectives therefore, must reflect the reason for the existence of the professions and their mission within the health services. The following set of objectives seeks to articulate those expectations and reasons for existence.

In the context of the current reform of the health services in Ireland, it is possible to identify three overarching objectives for nursing and midwifery:

1. Improving the quality of care provided to patients and clients
2. Improving access to care for patients and clients
3. Ensuring the capacity to deliver timely and effective health care services.

The achievement of these overarching objectives implies a further set of objectives for nursing and midwifery:

- To act as the principal coordinator of care on behalf of the patient or client and to ensure that the care provided is focused on the needs of the individual in both primary and acute settings.
- To expand the scope of practice of nursing and midwifery in a manner that is responsive to the needs of patients and clients and enhances the contribution of nursing and midwifery to the achievement of health care outcomes. This will include the management of patient and client caseloads and the development of nurse-/midwife-led clinics, involving generalist nurses and midwives, CNSs/CMSs and ANPs/AMPs as appropriate.
- To enhance the levels of cooperation between nursing and midwifery and other health care professionals and support workers in the context of multidisciplinary teams.
- To increase the presence of nursing and midwifery in the community based on health need. This implies a patient-centred, health-focused, holistic nursing orientation to practice that is complementary to existing models of care delivery. It is not based on physician replacement, but on health need. It may involve providing alternatives to physician-based services and may avoid the need for patients and clients to have access to physicians or acute services.
- To promote a positive understanding of health and approaches to healthy living in patients, clients, their families and communities. This involves providing advice,

information and education and is focused on empowering the individual to manage their own care and well-being.

The achievement of these objectives will serve to meet the expectations and requirements of the key stakeholders within the health services and will ensure that the specific contribution of nursing and midwifery to the development of the health care services of the future is maximised.

Key Strategies

This section will identify and provide an outline of the six key strategies that need to be put in place to achieve the objectives of nursing and midwifery within the health care services while taking advantage of the strengths of the professions, tackling the weaknesses, exploiting the opportunities and minimising the threats.

1. **Provide strategic coordination and leadership for the professions of nursing and midwifery.**
   This includes:
   - Devising ways to fill the leadership gap that exists within the professions
   - Building mechanisms for coordination and communication across the professions
   - Building professional identity for nursing and midwifery
   - Promoting innovative approaches to professional development
   - Promoting the use of joint appointments
   - Devising innovative ways of communicating with staff nurses and midwives to promote and deepen their understanding of the essence of nursing and midwifery.
2. **Contribute to the integration of health care services in cooperation with other health care professionals and support workers.**
   This includes:
   - Promoting and actively cooperating in initiatives aimed at increasing the integration of services at national, regional and local levels
   - Promoting an understanding within the services of the role that nursing and midwifery can play in achieving greater integration of services

- Promoting nursing and midwifery participation in multidisciplinary teams in acute and primary care settings
- Developing posts within service plans for appointments that span the boundaries between acute and primary care services.

3. **Devise and implement national, regional and local skill mix development plans.**
   This includes:

   - Building awareness and understanding of how skill mix initiatives can contribute to improving the quality and efficiency of care in different care settings
   - Developing channels of communication with regulatory bodies and representative associations of other health care professionals and support workers to promote innovative approaches to skill mix.

4. **Develop nursing and midwifery services.**
   This includes:

   - Identifying priority service development areas in partnership with service managers at national, regional and local levels
   - Promoting an understanding of how nursing-/midwifery-led services can contribute to the quality and efficiency of the services
   - Supporting initiatives in primary and acute services for the development of services, either led by nurses and midwives, or with nurse and midwife participation, as appropriate
   - Cooperating with other health care professionals and support workers in the development of appropriate services at national, regional and local level.

5. **Build nursing and midwifery capacity in the community.**
   This includes:

   - Cooperating with national, regional and local service managers in the identification of health needs that can be met by nurses and midwives working in the community
   - Engaging with national, regional and local service managers in mapping the areas in the community where the greatest need for a nursing and midwifery presence exists

- Developing nursing and midwifery follow-up services from acute health care settings, reaching out into the community and following up on patients´ needs
- Promoting within nursing and midwifery the concept of the nurse/midwife in the community
- Influencing the service planning process to ensure priority is given to increasing the presence of nurses and midwives in the community
- Encouraging a shift away from the provision of services in acute settings to the delivery of nurse-/midwife-led services in the community.

6. **Review and renew the strategic plan for the professional development of nursing and midwifery.**

    - This strategic plan requires initial discussion at a national level between key stakeholders in order to achieve buy-in. Thereafter, there would be regular reviews of this strategy, including a review of the priorities identified within it, in the light of changing circumstances within the health services and the changing needs of patients and clients.

CHAPTER 12

Strategic Actions

Action Programmes

In order to implement the strategies outlined in the previous chapter, it will be necessary for concerted action by the key stakeholders involved in the health services. The actions are summarised in Table 29.

Table 29: Action Programmes, Stakeholders and Indicators

Action programmes	Stakeholders	Measure of success
1. Provide strategic coordination and leadership for the professions of nursing and midwifery	• DoHC • HSE • ABA • National Council • Educational institutions • NMPDUs • Directors of nursing and midwifery	1. Action plans are in place to fill the leadership gap that exists within the professions. 2. Mechanisms for coordination and communication across the professions are being developed. 3. Professional identity of nursing and midwifery is being promoted through a series of strategic interventions. 4. Professional development for nurses and midwives is prioritised in service planning and policy. 5. Joint appointments are evident throughout the professions. 6. The essence of nursing and midwifery is being promoted through a series of strategic communications exercised with the professions.
2. Contribute to the integration of healthcare services in cooperation with other	• HSE • National Council • NMPDUs • Directors of nursing and midwifery	1. Strategic action plans are agreed to promote the integration of services at national, regional and local levels. 2. Communications plans are in place throughout the services to

Table 29: (*Continued*)

Action programmes	Stakeholders	Measure of success
healthcare professionals and support workers		promote the role that nursing and midwifery can play in achieving greater integration of services. 3. Nationwide plans are in place to build nursing and midwifery participation in multidisciplinary teams in acute and primary care settings. 4. Service plans make provision for making appointments that span the boundaries between acute and primary care services.
3. Devise and implement national, regional and local skill mix development plans	• DoHC • HSE • National Council • NMPDUs • Directors of nursing and midwifery	1. Communications, training and development plans are in place aimed at building awareness and understanding of how skill mix initiatives can contribute to improving the quality and efficiency of care in different care settings. 2. Detailed discussions are taking place with regulatory bodies and representative associations of other healthcare professionals and support workers to promote innovative approaches to skill mix.
4. Develop nursing and midwifery services	• HSE • National Council • Educational institutions • NMPDUs • Directors of nursing and midwifery	1. Priority service development areas are being identified in partnership with service managers at national, regional and local levels. 2. Communications, training and development initiatives are in place aimed at promoting an understanding of how nursing-/midwifery-led services can contribute to the quality and efficiency of the services. 3. Service plans provide for the support of initiatives in primary and acute services for the development of services, either led by nurses and midwives, or with nurse and midwife participation, as appropriate. 4. Cooperation with other healthcare professionals and support workers

Table 29: (*Continued*)

Action programmes	Stakeholders	Measure of success
		in the development of appropriate services at national, regional and local levels.
5. Build nursing and midwifery capacity in the community	• HSE • National Council • Educational institutions • NMPDUs • Directors of nursing and midwifery	1. Cooperation mechanisms exist with national, regional and local service managers in the identification of health needs that can be met by nurses and midwives working in the community. 2. Nurses and midwives engage with national, regional and local service managers in mapping the areas in the community where the greatest need for a nursing and midwifery presence exists. 3. Nursing and midwifery follow-up services from acute healthcare settings, reaching out into the community and following up on patient needs, are developed. 4. Strategic communications and promotion exercises exist to promote within nursing and midwifery the concept of the nurse/midwife in the community. 5. Service plans give priority to increasing the presence of nurses and midwives in the community. 6. Incentives exist to encourage a shift away from the provision of services in acute settings to the delivery of nurse- and midwife-led services in the community.
6. Review and renew the strategic plan for the professional development of nursing and midwifery	• DoHC • HSE • ABA • National Council • Educational institutions • NMPDUs • Directors of nursing and midwifery	1. This strategic plan requires initial discussion at national level between key stakeholders in order to achieve buy-in. Thereafter regular reviews of this strategy are required, including a review of the priorities identified within it, in the light of changing circumstances within the health services and the changing needs of patients and clients.

The Next Steps

The next steps in the process of making and implementing a strategy involve the generation of ownership of the implications and outcomes of the strategy devised on the basis of the present study. This will require detailed engagement with the leaders of the services, at executive and policy levels, and the creation of structures for coordination and communication within the professions. It will also require the dissemination of the messages of the research throughout the professions through publications, seminars, workshops and conferences. The adoption of this strategy will require further detailed negotiation and development in response to emerging changes and needs, some of which may be anticipated while others may not.

An important dimension of strategic planning is that of timing. It is important to have a clear timeframe for a strategy as this will provide a sense of purpose and will define the urgency with which tasks need to be tackled. With this in mind, the strategy for the professional development of nursing and midwifery should be implemented over a ten-year timeframe with review points throughout the period. The detailed indicators for each year need to be negotiated with the individual stakeholders. At the end of year three, it should be revised and a new five-year strategy devised. This should provide the opportunity for a rolling dynamic strategic development process to be introduced into the planning and development of the professions in Ireland. This dynamic approach is required in order to adapt to the changes that will occur at a fast pace within the health services. Details of the timing of specific elements of the strategy will be the subject of the negotiation and development involved in the next steps.

This research and the strategy based upon it do not pretend to be complete. By its very nature, and by the nature of the ongoing reform and transformation of health services in Ireland, the strategy needs to be constantly reviewed, revised and updated with reference to any future research, policy or ideological change. It is, however, an important step along the way to building a future for the professions of nursing and midwifery within a changing health service that takes advantage of the richness of the talents already available within the professions to shape the role the professions can play. But that future should not be perceived as being cast in stone; it should be perceived as evolving and developing, adapting and changing.

Endnotes

Preface

1. Commission on Nursing (1998).
2. Department of Health and Children (2005a).

Chapter 1: The Essence of Nursing

3. Nightingale (1860).
4. Henderson (1961).
5. WHO (1996).
6. Kitson (1999).
7. e.g. Benner (1984); Titchen (1998).
8. Rogers (1976).
9. Kitson (1999).
10. Benner (1984); Benner et al. (1999).
11. Neuman (1995).
12. George (1996).
13. Benner (1984).
14. Orem (1985).
15. Roper, Logan and Tierney (2000).
16. Henderson (1966).
17. Laing (1971).
18. National Council (2007b, 2007c).

Chapter 2: Nursing and Midwifery in Ireland

19. An Bord Altranais (2007f).
20. Government of Ireland (1919).
21. Government of Ireland (1950, 1961, 1985).
22. National Council (2003a).
23. An Bord Altranais (2007f).
24. Treacy and Hyde (2003).
25. ICM/WHO/FIGO (1992). The definition of a midwife was adopted by the International Confederation of Midwives (ICM), International Federation of Gynaecologists and Obstetricians (FIGO), in 1972 and 1973 respectively and later adopted by the World Health Organisation (WHO).

This definition was amended by the ICM in 1990 and the amendment ratified by the FIGO and the WHO in 1991 and 1992 respectively.

26. An Bord Altranais (2000a, p. 6).
27. Department of Health (1997b).
28. NEHB (2001).
29. Commission on Nursing (1998); An Bord Altranais (2001).
30. Community Midwifery Service, National Maternity Hospital (2001).
31. Department of Health (1984).
32. Sheridan (2000).
33. Expert Group on Mental Health Policy (2006).
34. Commission of Enquiry on Mental Handicap (1965).
35. Chavasse (2000).
36. An Bord Altranais (2007a).
37. Kelleher and Musgrave (2000).
38. National Council (2003a).
39. An Bord Altranais (2005a).
40. Hanafin et al. (2002).
41. National Council (2003a).
42. Hanafin et al. (2002).
43. National Council (2003a).
44. An Bord Altranais (2005a).
45. Labour Court (1997).
46. Commission on Nursing (1998) (see Chapter 1).
47. Government of Ireland (1985)
48. Cowan (1998).
49. Department of Health and Children (1999b).
50. St. James's Hospital (1996).
51. Working Party on General Nursing (1980).
52. National Council (2007a).
53. National Council (2006a).
54. Castledine (2003a).
55. An Bord Altranais (2000a).
56. Castledine (2003a).
57. National Council (2001b, 2004b, 2007c).
58. National Council (2002).
59. National Council (2005b).
60. National Council (2006b).

61. National Council (2007d).
62. National Council (2005c).
63. Begley et al. (2007).
64. National Council (2006c).
65. Department of Health and Children (2003d).
66. National Council (2005d).
67. Department of Health and Children (2001a).
68. National Task Force on Medical Staffing (2003).
69. Department of Health and Children (2003f).
70. Mid-Western Health Board (2003).
71. National Council (2004c).
72. National Council (2005e).
73. HSE (2006b).
74. National Council (2005f).
75. Department of Health (Britain) (2000).
76. An Bord Altranais (2000a).
77. An Bord Altranais (2001).
78. National Council (2004d).
79. National Council (2004d).
80. National Council (2005e).
81. National Council (2003a).
82. Department of Health and Children (2001a).
83. Prospectus Strategy Consultants (2003).
84. An Bord Altranais and the National Council (2005).
85. An Bord Altranais (2007a, 2007b, 2007c, 2007d, 2007e).
86. OHM (2000).
87. OHM (2003b).
88. OHM (2003c).
89. OHM (2004a).
90. OHM (2004b).
91. European Ministers of Education (1999).
92. An Bord Altranais (2005c).
93. *Irish Times* (2007e).
94. *Irish Times* (2007h).
95. Aiken et al. (2000).
96. HSE (2007f).
97. National Council (2003a, p. 7).
98. National Council (2004d); Medel-Anonuevo et al. (2001).

99. HSE (2007g).
100. National Council (2003b, 2006d).
101. National Council (2003a).
102. National Council (2004d).
103. National Council (2005a).
104. Leahy-Warren and Tyrrell (1998).
105. National Council (2005g).
106. Office for Public Management (2001).

Chapter 3: A Changing Society and its Implications for Nursing and Midwifery

107. Fahey et al. (2007).
108. ESRI (2008).
109. CSO (2007b).
110. CSO (2004a).
111. CSO (2006).
112. CSO (2006).
113. CSO (2006).
114. Data based on a number of sources.
115. HSE (2008a).
116. OECD (2007).
117. ESRI (2002).
118. ESRI (2002).
119. Department of Health and Children (2001a).
120. CSO (2007a).
121. Kelly et al. (2007); Barron and Kelly (2006).
122. CSO (2007a).
123. WHO (2004).
124. Friel et al. (1999).
125. Kelleher et al. (2003).
126. National Task Force on Obesity (2005).

Chapter 4: The Health Service Reform Programme

127. Department of Health and Children (2003a).
128. Prospectus Strategy Consultants (2003).
129. Commission on Financial Management and Control Systems in the Health Service (2003).
130. National Task Force on Medical Staffing (2003).
131. Department of Health and Children (2001a).
132. Government of Ireland (1994, 1997a); Department of the

Taoiseach (1996).
133. Barrington (1987).
134. O'Hara (1998).
135. Department of Health (1986).
136. WHO (1981).
137. Commission on Health Funding (1989).
138. Dublin Hospital Initiative Group (1991).
139. Department of Health (1994).
140. Department of Health (1997a).
141. Department of Health and Children (1998).
142. Government of Ireland (1997a).
143. Government of Ireland (1997b).
144. Prospectus Strategy Consultants (2003)
145. *Irish Times* (2007b).
146. Department of Health and Children (2003f).
147. Department of Health and Children (2003a).
148. Department of Health and Children (2005a).
149. HSE (2008b).
150. Department of Health and Children (2005b).
151. Government of Ireland (2007c).
152. iHIQA (2007).
153. Commission on Patient Safety and Quality Assurance (2008).
154. HSE (2006a).
155. *Irish Times* (2007g).
156. OHM (2003a).
157. Griffiths (1983).
158. Department of Health (Britain) (1989).
159. Department of Health (Britain) (1992).
160. Great Britain (1990).
161. OHM (2003a).
162. OHM (2003a).
163. Department of Health (Britain) (2000).
164. Department of Health (Britain) (1998).
165. Scanlan (2006).
166. HSE (2006b).
167. HSE (2006d).
168. PA Knowledge Ltd. (2007).
169. Teamwork Management Services Ltd (2006).

170. *Irish Times* (2007a).
171. HSE (2007c).
172. *Irish Times* (2007a).
173. *Irish Times* (2007b).
174. *Irish Times* (2007d).
175. *Irish Times* (2007c).
176. TIGER (2007).
177. HSE (2006c).
178. Cardiovascular Health Strategy Group (1999).
179. Department of Health and Children (2003b).
180. Department of Health and Children (2000).
181. National Advisory Committee on Palliative Care (2001).
182. Department of Tourism, Sport and Recreation (2001).
183. Department of Health and Children (2001b).
184. Department of Health (1988).
185. HSE (2008b).

Chapter 5: Two Key Issues in Strategic Planning

186. Nursing and Midwifery Resource Steering Group (2002).
187. Department of Health and Children (2002b).
188. DATHs (2000).
189. Aiken et al. (2000).
190. Aiken (1995).
191. Working Group on the Effective Utilisation of Professional Skills of Nurses and Midwives (2001).
192. Department of Health and Children (2001c).
193. Department of Health and Children (2003e).
194. <http://www.skillproject.ie>; FAS (2005).
195. Flynn (1998).
196. Department of Health and Children (2003c).
197. OHM (2000).
198. Kanter (1993).
199. Laschinger (2001).
200. Campbell (1987).
201. Aiken et al. (1994).
202. Laschinger et al. (1999).
203. Laschinger et al. (2001).
204. Irvine et al. (1999).
205. Klakovich (1995).

206. National Council (2001a).
207. National Council (2001b).
208. National Council (2002).
209. National Council (2004c).
210. National Council (2004a, 2004b).
211. National Council (2005e).
212. National Council (2001c).
213. National Council (2007e).
214. National Council (2003c).
215. National Council (2003b, 2006d).
216. National Council (2003a).
217. National Council (2004d).
218. National Council (2005f).
219. National Council (2005b).
220. National Council (2006b).
221. National Council (2007d).
222. National Council (2005c).
223. Kantor (1993).
224. Upenieks (2003).
225. Carney (2004).
226. Fradd (2004).
227. Sofarelli (1998).

Chapter 6: Learning from International Strategies for Nursing and Midwifery

228. WHO (1993).
229. WHO (1996).
230. WHO (1994).
231. WHO (1999).
232. WHO (2002).
233. Department of Health (Britain) (1999).
234. Scottish Executive Health Department (2001).
235. National Assembly for Wales (1999).
236. DHSSPS (2003).
237. DHSSPS/DoHC (2001, 2003, 2005).
238. DHSSPS (2004).
239. Department of Health (Britain) (2006).
240. Advisory Committee on Health Delivery and Human Resources (Canada) (2003).
241. Pan-Canadian Steering Committee (2005).

Chapter 8: Research Results: The Future of Health Services in Ireland

242. OHM (1998); OHM (2003d).

Chapter 9: Research Results: The Changing Role of Nursing and Midwifery

243. Benner (1984).
244. Commission on Nursing (1997).
245. WHO (2001).
246. National Council (2006f).
247. Scott et al. (2006).

Chapter 10: Research Results: Building Skills and Competencies

248. OHM (2000).
249. HSE (2007e, 2007f).
250. National Council (2006b).

Chapter 11: Strategic Issues for Nursing and Midwifery in Ireland

251. Expert Group on Mental Health Policy (2006).
252. An Bord Altranais (2000d).

Appendices

Appendix 1: List of Approved ANP/AMP Posts (October 2007)

AMP Posts Approved

AMP (Midwifery Care) x 1
AMP (Women's Health) x 1

ANP Posts Approved

ANP (Addiction and Mental Health) x 1
ANP (Breast Care) x 1
ANP (Cardiology) x 3
ANP (Cardiothoracic) x 9
ANP (Care of the Older Person) x 1
ANP (Child and Adolescent Mental Health and Psychotherapy) x 1
ANP (Children's Emergency) x 2
ANP (Children's Renal) x 1
ANP (Cognitive Behavioural Therapy) x 3
ANP (Colorectal) x 1
ANP (Community Older Adults) x 1
ANP (Diabetes) x 5
ANP (Eating Disorders) x 2
ANP (Emergency) x 46
ANP (Emergency Cardiology) x 2
ANP (Epilepsy) x 1
ANP (Gastroenterology) x 1
ANP (Haematology) x 2
ANP (Haematology Oncology) x 1
ANP (Heart Failure) x 1
ANP (Liaison Psychiatry) x 1
ANP (Neonatology) x 4
ANP (Occupational Health) x 1
ANP (Older Person with Dementia) x 2
ANP (Oncology) x 3
ANP (Pain Management) x 1

Appendix 1: (*Continued*)

ANP (Palliative Care) x 1
ANP (Primary Care) x 2
ANP (Rheumatology) x 2
ANP (Sexual Health) x 1
ANP (Specialist Palliative Care) x 3
ANP (Stroke Care) x 1
ANP (Tissue Viability) x 1
ANP (Urology) x 1
ANP (Women's Health) x 2
Total 113

Appendix 2: List of Approved CNS/CMS Posts (July 2008)

Title and Number of Posts	
Acute Mental Health	1
Acute Mental Health Care	2
Acute Pain Management	2
Addiction Counselling	26
Addiction Counsellor	24
Addictions	1
Addictions/Detoxification	2
Adolescent Mental Health	1
Adult Physical Disabilities and Rehabilitation	1
Adults with Autistic Spectrum Disorder	1
Adults with Chronic Physical Disabilities	1
Affective Disorders	5
Ageing Related Care	1
Airways Management	1
Airways/Tracheostomy	1
Alcohol Addiction Counselling	1
Alcohol Counselling	2
Alternative and Augmentative Communication	2
Alzheimer/Dementia Care	1
Anaesthetic Support	1
Anticoagulant	1
Apheresis	2
Art Therapy Interventions	1
Assertive Outreach Mental Health	1
Asthma	4
Asylum Seeker Health Assessment	1
Autism Hyperactive Disorder	1
Autism Therapist	2
Autistic Spectrum Disorders	1
Autotransfusion	3
Behaviour Management	8
Behaviour Nurse Challenging Behaviour Unit	1
Behaviour Nurse Psychotherapist	1
Behaviour Nurse Therapist	2

Appendix 2: (*Continued*)

Title and Number of Posts	
Behaviour Therapy	25
Behavioural Nurse Psychotherapist	1
Behavioural Psychotherapy	4
Behavioural Therapist	2
Behavioural Therapy	1
Bereavement	1
Bereavement and Loss	2
Bereavement Counselling	3
Bone Bank Coordinator	4
Bone Marrow Registry Coordination	1
Bone Marrow Transplant Coordinator	1
Bone Tumour	1
Brainwave Community, Epilepsy	1
Breast Care	23
Breastfeeding	1
Cancer Care	2
Cancer Coordinator	3
CAPD (Central Auditory Processing Disorders)	2
Cardiac Disease	1
Cardiac Disease Management	2
Cardiac Rehabilitation	27
Cardiac Services	4
Cardiology	10
Cardiology/Chest Pain	1
Cardio-Pulmonary Resuscitation	10
Cardio-Pulmonary Resuscitation – Neonatal	1
Care of the Elderly	1
Care of the Elderly – Learning Disabilities	1
Care of the Older Person	1
Challenging Behaviour	5
Challenging Behaviour Support	1
Chemotherapy	3
Chest Pain	7
Chest Pain Assessment	5

Appendix 2: (*Continued*)

Title and Number of Posts	
Child and Adolescent Mental Health	4
Child and Adolescent Psychiatry	5
Child and Adolescent Psychiatry Liaison	1
Child and Family Counselling	1
Child Psychiatry	1
Chronic Kidney Disease (Pre-Renal)	1
Chronic Renal Failure	1
Cognitive Behaviour Therapy	2
Cognitive Behavioural Psychotherapist	1
Cognitive Behavioural Therapy	4
Coloproctology	3
Colorectal	2
Colposcopy	5
Community Child and Adolescent Psychiatry	36
Community Early Services	1
Community Gerontology	1
Community Intellectual Disability	4
Community Intellectual Disability Nursing	5
Community Mental Handicap	16
Community Mental Health	24
Community Mental Health Nurse	207
Community Mental Health – Older Person	1
Community Paediatrics	1
Community Psychiatry of Old Age	9
Community Rehabilitation of the Older Person	1
Complementary Therapies	1
Complementary Therapy	4
Complementary/Supportive Therapies	1
Complementary/Supportive Therapies (Older Persons)	1
Consultation Liaison Psychiatry	1
Continence Advice	4
Continence Advisor	1
Continence Management Elderly Care Services	2

Appendix 2: (*Continued*)

Title and Number of Posts	
Continence Promotion	9
Continence Promotion in Learning Disabilities	2
Continence/Urodynamics	1
Continuous Ambulatory Peritoneal Dialysis	3
Counselling	10
Counselling and Psychotherapy	4
Counsellor	3
Creative, Diversional and Recreational Activation	10
Crisis Assessment and Treatment	2
Crisis Intervention	3
Crisis Intervention Liaison	1
Crisis Outreach Response	3
Critical Care	1
Cystic Fibrosis	16
Cystic Fibrosis Liaison	2
Deliberate Self-Harm	1
Dementia	3
Dementia Care	6
Dermatology	23
Diabetes	64
Diabetes – Community	1
Diabetes – Primary Care	1
Diabetes/Endocrine	2
Diabetes and Obesity	1
Diabetes Liaison	1
Diabetes Liaison – Primary Care	1
Diabetes Nurse Education	1
Diabetic Care	1
Disabilities	3
Diversional and Recreational Activation	1
Diversional and Recreational Activation for the Older Person	1
Diversional Therapy	2
Divisional Therapy/Health Promotion	1

Appendix 2: (*Continued*)

Title and Number of Posts	
DOMINO Early Discharge Team	3
Drama Therapy	1
Drug Court	1
Drugs Liaison	3
Dyspnoea	1
Early Intervention	16
Early Intervention – Autism	1
Early Intervention – Disabilities	2
Eating Disorders	3
Elderly Assessment	1
Elderly Care	1
Elderly Mentally Ill	1
Emergency Practice	3
Endocrine Liaison	1
Endocrine Nurse Specialist	1
Enduring Mental Illness	1
ENT (Ear, Nose and Throat)	1
ENT Assessment – Emergency Department	1
ENT/Head and Neck	2
Epidermolysis Bullosa Liaison	1
Epilepsy	4
Epilepsy and Health Promotion	1
Falls/Osteoporosis	2
Falls/Blackouts	2
Family and Marital Therapist	2
Family Therapist	8
Family Therapy	8
Family Therapy Nurse	1
Feeding and Nutrition	1
Foetal Assessment	7
Foetal Assessment and Ultrasonography	1
Functional Gerontology	1
Gastroenterology	3
General Practice	205

Appendix 2: (*Continued*)

Title and Number of Posts	
Genetics	1
Gerontological Assessment	1
Gerontology	5
Haematology	13
Haematology/Inherited Disorders of Coagulation	1
Haematology/Oncology	3
Haematology/Oncology in Parent Education	1
Haemoglobinopathy	2
Haemophilia	2
Haemophilia and Related Disorders	2
Haemovigilance	14
Haemovigilance and Blood Transfusion	1
Haemovigilance/Transfusion Surveillance	1
Head and Neck Oncology	2
Health and Well-Being	1
Health Advisor	4
Health Assessment and Promotion in the Older Adult	1
Health Promotion	1
Health Promotion and Intervention	4
Health Promotion and Intervention – Intellectual Disability Nursing	1
Health Promotion (Forensic)	2
Health Promotion and Intervention	1
Health Promotion for Ageing Adults with Intellectual Disability	1
Health Promotion in Intellectual Disabilities	1
Heart Efficiency	2
Heart Failure	10
Hepatitis C	1
Hepatitis C Liaison	3
Hepatitis C Research	1
Hepatology	8

Appendix 2: (*Continued*)

Title and Number of Posts	
Hepatology, Hepatitis C	1
HIV/AIDS Liaison	2
HIV/Infectious Diseases	2
Home-Based Mental Health Treatment	1
Home-Based Treatment – Acute Psychiatry	8
Homelessness Liaison	1
Ilizarov Method	2
Immunology	1
Infection Control	56
Infection Control/Occupational Health	1
Infectious Disease Liaison	1
Infectious Diseases	2
Integrative Counselling	3
Interventional Radiology	1
Invasive Cardiology	1
Joint Replacement	1
Lactation	14
Laser Therapy	1
Liaison (Self-Harm)	1
Liaison Mental Health	2
Liaison Psychiatry	5
Lithotripsy	1
Liver Transplant Coordinator	3
Lung Cancer	1
Lung Cancer Nursing	1
Lung Transplant Coordinator	1
Lymphodema	2
Male Genito-Urinary Cancer	1
Mammography	1
Mental Health Education	1
Mental Health in Adults with an Intellectual Disability	2
Mental Health Liaison	1

Appendix 2: (*Continued*)

Title and Number of Posts	
Mental Health Promotion	1
Mental Health Promotion and Intervention	1
Mental Health Rehabilitation	7
Metabolic Disorder	1
Migraine/Headache	1
Minor Injuries	1
Mobility and Therapeutic Interventions	1
Motor Neuron Disease Liaison	1
Multiple Sclerosis	3
Multiple Sclerosis/Neuro-Immunology	1
Neonatal	3
Neonatal and Paediatric Neurology	1
Neonatal Resuscitation	1
Neonatal Transition Home Service	1
Neonatology	1
Nephrology	3
Neurology	7
Neurology Liaison	1
Nutrition	1
Nutrition Support	1
Occupational Health	34
Old Age Psychiatry	2
Older People Nursing	2
Older Person Learning Disabilities	1
Oncology	46
Oncology Liaison	14
Oncology/Breast Care	1
Oncology/Palliative Care	1
Ophthalmology	12
Opthalmic Assessment – Emergency Department	2
Orthopaedic Casting and Splinting	6
Orthopaedics	2
Osteoporosis	1

Appendix 2: (*Continued*)

Title and Number of Posts	
Paediatric Casting	1
Paediatric Diabetes	4
Paediatric Ear, Nose and Throat	1
Paediatric Endocrinology	1
Paediatric Haemodialysis	1
Paediatric Liaison	3
Paediatric Link Nurse	1
Paediatric Neurology	2
Paediatric Oncology	1
Paediatric Oncology Liaison	2
Paediatric Opthalmology	1
Paediatric Orthopaedics	1
Paediatric Pain	1
Paediatric Pain Management	1
Paediatric Radiology	1
Paediatric Renal	1
Paediatric Respiratory	3
Pain Control	5
Pain Management	9
Pain Medicine	1
Palliative Care	79
Palliative Care – Learning Disabilities	1
Palliative Care Inpatient Unit	1
Palliative Home Care	137
Parasuicide/Deliberate Self-Harm	1
Parent Educator	1
Parkinson's Disease	1
Parkinson's Disease/Aspen	1
Peri-Anaesthesia	1
Peritoneal Dialysis	2
Personal Development Programmes	3
Physical and Mobility Habilitation	1
Physical Disability	1

Appendix 2: (*Continued*)

Title and Number of Posts	
Physical Disability with Special Needs	2
Plaster Care – Paediatric	1
Pre-Assessment	1
Pre-Operative Assessment	1
Pre-School Learning Disability and Autism	1
Primary Care	1
Primary Care (Mental Health)	1
Psychiatric Consultation Liaison	2
Psychiatry of Old Age	1
Psychiatry of Old Age – Dementia Care	1
Psycho-Oncology	1
Psychosis	2
Psychosocial Interventions	1
Psychotherapy	1
Psychotic Disorders	2
Rehabilitation – Mental Health	2
Rehabilitation Care of the Older Person	1
Rehabilitation Nursing	1
Renal	5
Renal – Pre-Transplant	1
Renal Anaemia	1
Renal Transplantation Services	1
Reproductive Health Care	2
Respiratory	29
Respiratory/Asthma	1
Respiratory Care	4
Respiratory Care, Sleep Disorders	2
Respiratory Medicine	1
Respiratory Nursing	1
Resuscitation	5
Rheumatology	16
School Children with Special Needs	1
Sensory Integration and Therapeutic Programmes	1

Appendix 2: (*Continued*)

Title and Number of Posts	
Serious and Enduring Mental Illness	1
Sexual Health Promotion	1
Sexual Health/AIDS Liaison	1
Smoking Cessation	4
Smoking Cessation/Health Promotion	1
Social and Vocational Rehabilitation	1
Specialist Palliative Care	3
Spinal Cord Injury – Liaison Nursing Service	1
Stem Cell	1
Stoma and Breast Care	1
Stoma Care	20
Stomatherapy	2
Stress Management/Bio-Feedback	1
Stroke Care	4
Stroke Management/Rehabilitation	1
Stroke Rehabilitation	1
Substance Misuse	2
Substance Misuse Counsellor	1
Supported Living	1
Surgical Liaison	1
Surgical Pre-Assessment Clinic	1
Systemic Family Therapy	2
Therapeutic Apheresis	1
Therapeutic Interventions in Elderly Care	1
Therapeutic Programmes	13
Therapies, Mental Health Care for Older People	1
Tissue Viability	24
Transfusion/Haemovigilance	1
Transfusion Surveillance	11
Transplant Liaison	1
Trauma and Minor Injuries	1
Treatment of Alcohol and Drug Use Disorders	1
Treatment Resistive Schizophrenia	1
Ultrasonography	4

Appendix 2: (*Continued*)

Title and Number of Posts	
Ultrasonography and Early Pregnancy Assessment	1
Ultrasound	4
Ultrasound and Foetal Assessment	4
Upper G.I. Cancer	1
Urodynamics	6
Urodynamics and Continence Promotion	1
Urodynamics/Rectal Manometry	1
Urology	8
Vascular	1
Vocational Rehabilitation	5
Wound Care	5
Wound Care/Tissue Viability	1
Young Person's Substance Misuse	1
Total	**1982**

Appendix 3: Types of Nurse-led/Midwife-led Service and Numbers of Years Established (2005)

Type of service	Years established
Adult tissue viability clinic	7
Adult pre-assessment day care	4
Adult renal transplantation services	2
Adult haemocromatosis services	2
Adult pre-admission elective orthopaedics	2
Admission/discharge planning	3–4
Advanced nurse practitioner – Accident & Emergence service	1
Alzheimer unit	3
Assessment and case management in day hospital	3
Asylum seekers	2
Behavioural therapy	10
Blood collection clinics	2
Bone densitometry estimation	3
Cardiac rehabilitation	5
Care of older person	34
Case management	4
Case manager home subvention	1–10
Child health screening	20–34
Cognitive behavioural therapy	5–8
Colposcopy services	10
Community alcohol and substance misuse counselling services	7–8
Community midwifery	6
Community programme (mental health)	18
Continence assessment and management	4–28
Continuing care	Not specified
Convalescence care	3–15
Day care services	8–20
Deliberate self-harm liaison nurse	2
Dementia care services	6

Appendix 3: (*Continued*)

Type of service	Years established
Developing care plans	4
Diabetes	3
Disability service – assessment of needs	34
Ear irrigation	5
Early transfer home scheme	2
Extended care	20
Family therapy services	4
Foetal assessment	4
Generic counsellor: day services	3
Haemodialysis treatment	9
Heart failure	2–3
Home care	15
Hospice day care	11
Lactation	5
Leg ulcer clinic	1–4
Lymphoedema clinic	7
Midwife-led clinic	6
Midwifery-led unit	6 months
Midwives' clinics	15
Minor injuries A&E	3
Occupational health	5
Oncology services	3
Outreach clinics	3
Paediatric cystic fibrosis clinic	14
Paediatric/adult diabetes services	4–5
Paediatric/adult dermatology	7–12
Paediatric endocrinology	9
Paediatric respiratory services	7
Paediatric urology	7
Palliative care	1–14
Parent craft classes	6–25
Patient assessment	4
Postnatal care	15

Appendix 3: (*Continued*)

Type of service	Years established
Primary care wound clinic	5
Rehabilitation services	2
Residential services	50
Respiratory nurse clinic	3
Respite care	3–10
Respite care (crisis)	8
Respite care (planned)	8
School screening	34
School service	20–30
Substance abuse service	Not supplied
Therapeutic aphaeresis service	8 months
Travellers' service	10
Urodynamics	3
Women's health – practice nursing	1–6
Wound care including leg ulcer management – practice nursing	1–6

Note: Where the years are in multiples, more than one service provides this care; the range of years established are given.

Appendix 4: Types of Services that Directors of Nursing/Midwifery are Intending to Introduce in the Future

Reality and cognitive behavioural sessions with self-referral to a nurse-led community service
Day care service for older people
Rheumatology
ANP in pain management
Out-patient cataract nurse-led clinic
Incontinence care in the older person
Health promotion in the elderly
Nurse-led pre-admission assessment service
Challenging behaviour
Holistic assessment of clients in the community who may require elderly care
Nurse-led clinic for clients with enduring mental health difficulties
Nurse-led liaison service (mental health)
Nurse-led community detoxification programme
Diabetic ANP
Nurse-led colposcopy clinic
Midwife-led early miscarriage clinic
Midwife-led admissions and discharges
Tissue viability
Nurse-led pain management
Midwifery-led clinics
Pre-/post-HIV testing sessions
Nurse-led palliative care via ANP posts
Nurse-led care and case management (community care)
Nurse-led falls clinic
Nurse-led therapeutic day hospital
Midwifery-led ultrasonography service
Midwifery-led postnatal clinics
Midwifery-led breast-feeding support groups
Nurse-led mental health promotion
Nurse-led mental health rehabilitation
Nurse-led cognitive behavioural psychotherapy
Review of home birth services

Appendix 4: (*Continued*)

Eating, drinking and swallowing nurse-led clinic
Nurse-led glaucoma clinic
Nurse-led therapeutic apheresis
Nurse-led platelet apheresis
ANP radiation-induced toxicities
Midwifery-led services for healthy women likely to have a normal pregnancy and labour
Nurse-led child health primary screening
Nurse-led cervical cytology clinics
Nurse-led community leg ulcer clinics
Nurse-led enuresis treatment clinic
Nurse-led child health service

Appendix 5: Commission on Nursing – Summary of Progress

1. **Regulation of the Professions**
    - The recommendations in Chapter 4 of the *Report of the Commission on Nursing* (Regulation of the Profession) are being addressed in the context of the Nurses and Midwives (Amendment) Bill, 2007.
    - The health care assistants' programme was rolled out in 2003.
2. **Preparation for the Professions**
    - Nursing degree in general, psychiatric and intellectual disability nursing was introduced in 2002.
    - Eighteen centres for nurse education/centres for midwife education have been established.
    - The nursing career centre was established to promote nursing and midwifery as a career.
    - Forty sponsorships for mature student applications available annually.
3. **Professional Development**
    - The National Council for the Professional Development of Nursing and Midwifery was established in 1999.
    - Clinical career pathway framework of generalist, specialist and advanced practice has been established.
    - Frameworks for the establishment of clinical nurse/ midwife specialist posts and advanced nurse/midwife practitioner posts have been developed.
    - Roles including core concepts have been defined.
    - Eight nursing and midwifery planning and development units (NMPDUs) have been established.
    - Part of the role of the NMPDU includes overseeing the provision of continuing nursing and midwifery education for a health area.
    - Joint appointment between the Health Research Board and the National Council established for the promotion of research within nursing and midwifery.
    - Nursing research strategy published in 2003 and research committee established.

4. **The Role of Nurses and Midwives in the Management of Services**

    - A chief nursing officer was appointed in 1998 to the Department of Health and Children.
    - The role of the chief nursing officer includes playing a crucial role in the central planning and strategic development of nursing and midwifery and strengthening the workforce planning, professional leadership and quality assurance functions in the Department.
    - The *Nursing and Midwifery Resource: Final Report of the Steering Group Towards Workforce Planning* was published in 2002.
    - Two supporting texts were published relating to the study: *Guidance for Best Practice on the Recruitment of Overseas Nurses and Midwives* was published in December 2001 and the *Report of the National Study of Turnover in Nursing and Midwifery* was published in 2002.
    - NMPDUs were established in each health area, with a strategic planning and policy development role. It was intended that the directors of NMPDUs should operate at a strategic planning level.
    - The Commission defined the role of senior nursing and midwifery management as being to provide strategic and clinical leadership and direction for nursing and midwifery and related services. In order to emphasise this role, the title of all matrons in large acute hospitals and chief nursing officers in psychiatric services was changed to director of nursing.
    - Matrons of smaller hospitals (bands 3, 4 and 5) were to combine a professional development role with detailed management responsibilities and should be given more explicit involvement in the determination of the budget and greater control and responsibility over its utilisation. The implementation of this recommendation varies throughout the country.
    - The Commission recommended that middle nursing and midwifery management should have a defined management role and not merely a 'gatekeeping' administrative

function. The implementation of this recommendation varies throughout the country.

- The Commission recommended that first-line nursing and midwifery management should fulfil the following functions: professional clinical leadership; staffing and staff development; resource management; and facilitating communication. Management skills training was to be given. In recognition of these roles and of the differences in institutional settings in which first-line nursing and midwifery management works, a new grading structure and title changes have been introduced: clinical nurse manager 1 or clinical midwife manager 1 (reporting to a clinical nurse or midwife manager 2); clinical nurse manager 2 or clinical midwife manager 2 (in charge of a ward or unit area); and clinical nurse manager 3 or clinical midwife manager 3 (in charge of a department).

5. **Nursing and Midwifery in the Community**

- National strategy for nursing and midwifery in the community (NAMIC) steering group overseeing the development of the strategy met on thirteen occasions between November 2001 and October 2003. A final draft report which included template and action plan was discussed. The report has not been published.
- In 2004, the requirement for midwifery qualification for entry to the public health nurse diploma was removed and substituted by a module in maternity and childcare.
- The title superintendent public health nurse has been changed to director of public health nursing; the title senior public health nurse has been changed to assistant director public health nursing.
- Registered general nurses/midwives as part of the community nursing team are in place, with ongoing developments.
- To enhance the delivery of intellectual disability nursing services, twenty-three community intellectual disability clinical nurse specialists are in place with more in development.
- To ensure an enhanced community mental health nursing service, 252 community mental health clinical nurse special-

ists and one advanced nurse practitioner are in place, with more in development.

- Practice nurse coordinators have been established in each health area and are attached to the NMPDU, to assist in supporting the development needs of practice nurses.

6. **Nursing in Care of the Elderly**

- Nurse advisor/palliative care post was established in the Department of Health and Children in 2002.
- Regional practice development coordinators in care of older persons are attached to the NMPDU, responsible for the development of guidelines and policies for acute, community and nursing homes.
- Forty-six clinical nurse specialists and one advanced nurse practitioner in care of older person have been established.
- Centres of nurse education have completed a needs analysis of training needs for nurses working in care of the older person. Short education programmes are in place.

7. **Midwifery**

- A direct entry degree programme in midwifery commenced in 2006.

8. **Children's Nursing**

- In 2004, the title 'sick children's nurse' was replaced with the title 'registered children's nurse' (RCN).
- A direct entry degree programme in registered children's nursing/general nursing commenced in 2006.

Appendix 6: Policy Initiatives, Reports and Publications of the National Council – 2001 to 2008

Year/Initiative/Report/Publication	Summary
2001	
Criteria and Process for the Allocation of Additional Funding for Continuing Education (February)	This document outlines the criteria and processes involved in the allocation of additional funding for continuing professsional development and education for nurses and midwives.
Clinical Nurse/Midwife Specialists – Intermediate Pathway (April)	This document outlines the process for establishment of CNS/CMS posts and the criteria that nurses and midwives must meet in order to become CNSs/CMSs.
Framework for the Establishment of Advanced Nurse Practitioner and Advanced Midwife Practitioner Posts (May)	This document provides a definition of the role of ANP/AMP and defines the criteria that nurses and midwives must meet to in order to become ANPs/AMPs.
National Council Newsletter, Issues 1 to 4	The newsletter of the National Council was introduced in 2001 and is intended as a platform for the dissemination of information and analysis of issues of relevance to nurses and midwives in Ireland.
2002	
Guidelines on the Development of Courses Preparing Nurses and Midwives as Clinical Nurse/Midwife Specialists and Advanced Nurse/Midwife Practitioners (May)	This document was produced to assist providers of continuing/post-registration education programmes for CNSs/CMSs and for ANPs/AMPs. It provides guidelines in relation to development, design and evaluation of programmes.

Appendix 6: (*Continued*)

Year/Initiative/Report/Publication	Summary
National Council Newsletter, Issues 5 to 8	The newsletter continued to provide information on developments of relevance to nursing and midwifery in Ireland. In this year a detailed series of analyses on the implications of the Health Service Reform Programme was introduced aimed at familiarising nurses and midwives with the details and implications of the reform programme.
2003	
Agenda for the Future Professional Development of Nursing and Midwifery (May)	A consultation process was carried out nationally from March 2002 to March 2003. Workshops were held with directors of nursing and midwifery, directors of the NMPDUs, and nurses and midwives from all divisions of the register. Submissions were called for and 105 were received. The report benchmarks progress to date for general, midwifery, mental health, children's, intellectual disability and older person nursing and sets the agenda for a debate on options, direction and actions for the future. CPD emerges as the predominant issue in this report for all areas of nursing to support developing nursing and midwifery practice in modern health structures.
Guidelines for Portfolio Development for Nurses and Midwives (September)	These guidelines are aimed at individual nurses and midwives working at the forefront of health care delivery,

Appendix 6: (*Continued*)

Year/Initiative/Report/Publication	Summary
	for the purpose of assisting them to identify, reflect upon and record the contribution they make to direct and indirect care, encouraging them to store records of their development in a coherent and structured manner and providing guidance and information on achieving their individual professional goals within the context of the needs of the health service.
Guidelines for Health Service Providers for the Selection of Nurses and Midwives who might Apply for Financial Support in Seeking Opportunities to Pursue Further Education (November)	This document was produced to assist managers of health services in the selection of individuals seeking financial support to pursue further education and professional development.
National Council Newsletter, Issues 9 to 12	The newsletter continued to disseminate and analyse information of relevance to the profession, in particular detailed explanation and analysis of the Health Service Reform Programme was featured.
2004	
An Evaluation of the Effectiveness of the Role of the Clinical Nurse/Midwife Specialist (January)	This report benchmarks the progress of clinical specialism in nursing and midwifery in Ireland to the present time. Ireland is at an early stage of development of these roles within a formalised framework as set out by the *Report of*

Appendix 6: (*Continued*)

Year/Initiative/Report/Publication	Summary
	the Commission on Nursing. The cohorts of CNSs/CMSs in post have clearly embraced the core concepts of the role and have been empowered to improve the quality of care for patients/clients: there is overwhelming support for the effectiveness of the role of the CNS/CMS. It is clear that there is great potential for the role to develop in its responsiveness to service need. This report outlines critical areas for progress and describes a process for future development of roles at local, regional and national levels. The report makes recommendations regarding role development, continuing professional development, development of posts and annual reviews of posts on a local, regional and national basis.
Report on the Continuing Professional Development of Staff Nurses and Staff Midwives (May)	There is growing evidence of the need to link CPD with organisational goals. This report examines CPD issues relevant to staff nurses and staff midwives by reviewing CPD activities of staff nurses and midwives, competency achievement and maintenance relevant to service need, personal professional development of staff nurses and staff midwives, career choices relevant to CPD and competency of staff nurses and staff midwives. In preparation for this

Appendix 6: (*Continued*)

Year/Initiative/Report/Publication	Summary
	report methodology included a literature review, focus groups and questionnaires. Staff nurses from general, mental health, intellectual disability and children's nursing and staff midwives were invited to participate. Nurses and midwives from cities, towns and rural areas were represented, as were those working in community and in-patient settings. Recommendations are made concerning the development of structures to support CPD for staff nurses and staff midwives.
Framework for the Establishment of Advance Nurse and Advanced Midwife Practitioner Posts (Second Edition) (July)	This document, building on the framework outlined in the first edition, outlines the background to the development of ANP/AMP posts in Ireland. It defines ANP/AMP roles and outlines the criteria that nurses and midwives must meet in order to become ANPs/AMPs. It also provides guidance for managers, nurses and midwives who are working through the processes. Templates are provided to assist in the application processes.
Framework for the Establishment of Clinical Nurse/Midwife Specialist Posts (Second Edition) (November)	This document, building on the 2001 edition, outlines the process for establishment of CNS/CMS posts and the criteria that nurses and midwives must meet in order to become CNSs/CMSs. Core competencies for CNS posts are provided.

Appendix 6: (*Continued*)

Year/Initiative/Report/Publication	Summary
National Council Newsletter, Issues 13 to 15	The newsletter continued to be used as a platform for the dissemination and analysis of information relevant to the development of nursing and midwifery within the Health Services. In particular, detailed analysis of the HSRP continued.
NCNM Quarterly Review, Issue 16	The information and analysis in the newsletter developed to the point that it was decided to rebrand the newsletter as the *NCNM Quarterly Review*.
2005	
An Evaluation of the Extent and Nature of Nurse-Led/Midwife-Led Services in Ireland (April)	The terms of reference for the study were to examine the literature pertaining to the nurse-led/midwife-led care services, to identify the extent of nurse-led/midwife-led care services in Ireland and to make recommendations on future areas for developments for nurse-led/midwife-led care in Ireland. The methodology employed consisted of focus groups, questionnaires and a literature review. The diversity and multiplicity of the nurse-/midwife-led services in place would suggest that nurses and midwives are able to respond to patient/client need in a flexible and appropriate manner, allowing the development to occur within a multidisciplinary context. To date these initiatives

Appendix 6: (*Continued*)

Year/Initiative/Report/Publication	Summary
	have been driven by service need and a desire by nurses and midwives, both at senior and clinical level, to improve the quality of the patient/client care. It is also evident that as these services develop they are being audited and measured for clinical effectiveness and patient satisfaction. It is recommended that a business plan approach is adopted to aid the development of nurse-led/midwife-led services – a template to assist this is provided.
Clinical Nurse Specialist and Advanced Nurse Practitioner Roles in Emergency Departments: A Position Paper (April)	This position paper reviews progress of specialist and advanced practice in emergency departments to date, identifies key components of role development for specialist and advanced nursing practice within an emergency context and outlines the areas that require further development in order to enhance service. A focused needs assessment for managers is provided.
Agenda for the Future Professional Development of Public Health Nursing (June)	A consultation was carried out nationally from November 2004 to February 2005. Workshops were held with directors of public health nursing, assistant directors of public health nursing, public health nurses engaged in clinical practice and key stakeholders. The report benchmarks progress to date and sets an agenda for future actions. The main

Appendix 6: (*Continued*)

Year/Initiative/Report/Publication	Summary
	concerns expressed by participants related to role clarity, workload demands, variation in service provision and delivery of care, the clinical career pathway, leadership, skill mix and multidisciplinary team working. The report sets an agenda for future actions.
A Study to Identify the Research Priorities for Nursing and Midwifery in Ireland (June)	Under the national research strategy for nursing and midwifery in Ireland, a study to identify research priorities was carried out under the auspices of the National Council. The report was compiled by a team of researchers from UCD, led by Dr Therese Meehan.
Review of Nurses and Midwives in the Prescribing and Administration of Medicinal Products – Final Report (June, jointly with An Bord Altranais)	This report is the culmination of a three-and-a-half year project conducted jointly by the National Council and An Bord Altranais. The report includes an updated literature review, legislative issues, policy developments, activity trail, education programme, current health care policy and recommendations. The report identified the need for nurses and midwives in Ireland to expand their medication management practices to include prescribing medications where appropriate.
Review of Nurses and Midwives in the Prescribing and Administration of	This document provides a summary of the main report.

Appendix 6: (*Continued*)

Year/Initiative/Report/Publication	Summary
Medicinal Products – Summary (June, jointly with An Bord Altranais)	
The Development of Joint Appointments: A Framework for Irish Nursing and Midwifery (September)	This document provides guidance in the form of a framework for institutions and individuals involved in making joint appointments between services, voluntary organisations, educational institutions and/or other organisations. The report provides an overview of national and international literature and experiences. The need for clear structures and supports are identified as critical success factors. The National Council has created a framework assisting those involved in planning such roles.
Service Needs Analysis for Clinical Nurse/Midwife Specialists and Advanced Nurse/Midwife Practitioner Posts (September)	This paper identifies factors necessary for a service to conduct a needs analysis to determine whether specialist or advanced practice levels of nursing/midwifery practice are required to deliver a high quality service. A business case template is provided.
Preliminary Evaluation of the Role of the Advanced Nurse Practitioner (September)	This report shows that the roles have been successful where they have been introduced. The roles are spread over a wide variety of care areas, indicating that roles have developed in response to health service need. The strong clinical focus of the ANP role identified in the study

Appendix 6: (*Continued*)

Year/Initiative/Report/Publication	Summary
	suggests that one of the original aims of the Commission on Nursing, namely the retention of expert nurses in direct patient care, has been met.
NCNM Quarterly Review, Issue 17 to 20	The *Quarterly Review* continued to be used as a platform for the analysis and dissemination of information of relevance to the profession in the context of developments within the health services.
2006	
Guidelines for Portfolio Development for Nurses and Midwives (Second Edition) (February)	These guidelines are aimed at individual nurses and midwives working at the forefront of health care delivery, for the purpose of assisting them to identify, reflect upon and record the contribution they make to direct and indirect care, encouraging them to store records of their development in a coherent and structured manner and providing guidance and information on achieving their individual professional goals within the context of the needs of the health service. This publication provides an update on the original document published by the National Council in 2003. The document provides fourteen sample record sheets and is accompanied by a CD containing

Appendix 6: (*Continued*)

Year/Initiative/Report/Publication	Summary
	Microsoft Word versions of the record sheets and an Adobe Acrobat PDF version of the guidelines.
Report on the Baseline Survey of Research Activity in Irish Nursing and Midwifery (February)	This report provides a picture of nursing and midwifery research activity in Ireland for the period December 2002 to December 2004. A number of recommended actions support the recommendations of the national research strategy for nursing and midwifery in Ireland (p. 9). Other recommendations are set out for building upon the baseline established by this project.
A Guide to Sharing Practice and Quality Developments with Other Colleagues (June)	This publication is intended to help nurses and midwives prepare details of practice and quality developments for inclusion on the National Council's all-Ireland online practice and quality database.
Measurement of Nursing and Midwifery Interventions: Guidance and Resource Pack (September)	This is a two-part document. Part one contains a report on a study of nursing and midwifery interventions and the measurement of their outcomes taking place in Ireland. Part two contains the guidance and resource pack, which aims to assist nurses, midwives and services to select and assess nursing and midwifery interventions as part of a quality improvement initiative. A CD containing Adobe Acrobat PDF versions of the two books accompanies the document.

Appendix 6: (*Continued*)

Year/Initiative/Report/Publication	Summary
Improving the Patient Journey: Understanding Integrated Care Pathways (September)	This publication aims to promote the use of integrated care pathways by nurses and midwives in order to improve the patient's journey.
NCNM Quarterly Review, Issues 21 to 24	The *Quarterly Review* continued to be used as a platform for the analysis and dissemination of information of relevance to the profession in the context of developments within the health services.
2007	
Framework for the Establishment of Advanced Nurse Practitioner and Advanced Midwife Practitioner Posts (Third Edition) (February)	The third edition of the *Framework* was informed by the National Council's accumulated experience in handling advanced nurse/midwife practitioner post applications, the preliminary evaluation of the established roles, consultation with key stakeholders and developments taking place as part of the Health Service Reform Programme.
Framework for the Establishment of Clinical Nurse/Midwife Specialist Posts – Intermediate Pathway (Third Edition) (April)	The three most significant points in this third edition are the requirements for: • The clinical nurse/midwife specialist post-holder to have undertaken formal recognised post-registration education at Level 8 or above on the National Framework of Qualifications of the National Qualifications Authority of Ireland.

Appendix 6: (*Continued*)

Year/Initiative/Report/Publication	Summary
	• The employing organisation to give details of the essential qualifications, experience and competencies to fulfil the role and functions of the post. • An applicant for a clinical nurse/midwife specialist post to demonstrate that they have the competencies necessary to fulfil the job description.
Clinical Nurse Specialist and Advanced Nurse Practitioner Roles in Older Persons Nursing: Position Paper No. 3 (April)	Building on the existing clinical nurse specialist and advanced nurse practitioner frameworks, the service need analysis template (2005) and the previous position papers (2005 and 2006), this position paper on clinical nurse specialist and advanced nurse practitioner roles in older person services aims to provide guidance to the relevant service providers where the introduction of such posts is being considered. Key practice areas in which clinical nurse specialist posts relating to the nursing care of the older person have been established include Alzheimer's disease, dementia, community psychiatry of old age and rehabilitation of the older person, but service providers are advised to consider demographic trends, epidemiological factors, and health service policy when ascertaining the need for further posts.

Appendix 6: (*Continued*)

Year/Initiative/Report/Publication	Summary
Criteria and Processes for the Allocation of Additional Funding for Continuing Education (Second Edition) (June)	In light of the National Council's accumulated experience of processing applications for continuing education funding and 'best practice in funding' developments elsewhere, a decision was taken to allocate funding to three types of programme: short continuing education programmes (i.e. programmes that can be completed within twelve months), continuing education programme grants (i.e. programmes that may be of up to three years duration and pertain to specific strategic developments), and grants for advanced nurse/midwife practitioner post development (i.e. funding of a part-time facilitator to prepare a site and job description for an advanced nurse/midwife practitioner post). The revised *Criteria and Processes* clearly state the criteria for the three types of programme, as well as clarifying funding conditions and rules, and providing directions on how to make and submit an application for funding.
The Introduction of Nurse and Midwife Prescribing in Ireland: An Overview (September) (with the Health Service Executive, Department of Health and Children, and An Bord Altranais)	The National Council, in collaboration with the HSE, the Department of Health and Children, and An Bord Altranais, prepared this overview of the nurse and midwife prescribing in Ireland. Published in the same year as the relevant legislation, this document depicts the context in

Appendix 6: (*Continued*)

Year/Initiative/Report/Publication	Summary
	which prescriptive authority for nurses and midwives was achieved (subject to specific conditions), as well as demonstrating the need for this prescriptive authority within any modern health service. The legislative framework for nurse and midwife prescribing is outlined, and the respective roles of the key partners in the prescribing initiative are described. It is envisaged that this *Introduction* will be a useful reference and resource for the health service as a whole, as well as for nurses and midwives of all grades.
NCNM *Quarterly Review*, Issues 25 to 28	The *Quarterly Review* continued to be used as a platform for the analysis and dissemination of information of relevance to the profession in the context of developments within the health services.
2008	
Framework for the Establishment of Advanced Nurse Practitioner and Advanced Midwife Practitioner Posts (Fourth Edition) (January)	The fourth edition of the *Framework* relating to the preparation of sites for ANPs/AMPs remains unchanged, as do the criteria and templates for applications, job descriptions and financial approval for posts.
Accreditation of Advanced Nurse Practitioners and Advanced Midwife Practitioners (Fourth Edition) (January)	Details relating to the accreditation of ANPs/AMPs are now published in a separate companion document. The criteria for accreditation by the National Council are unaltered

Appendix 6: (*Continued*)

Year/Initiative/Report/Publication	Summary
	except for the insertion of some explanatory notes. Some minor amendments have been made to the guidance for re-accreditation of ANPs/AMPS.
Enhanced Nursing Practice in Emergency Departments: Position Paper No. 4 (April)	Building upon its first position paper (*Clinical Nurse Specialist and Advanced Nurse Practitioner Roles*, April 2005) as well as *Service Needs Analysis for Clinical Nurse/Midwife Specialist and Advanced Nurse/Midwife Practitioner Posts* (September 2005) and accumulated experience in developing the clinical career pathway in order to provide clear and explicit guidance so as to develop nursing roles within emergency departments in Irish hospitals, this guidance is set in the context of the evidence from these emergency departments and the educational programmes provided by the third level education sector in response to service need. This document provides a framework for determining the need for enhanced nursing roles and elaborated on matters relating to scope of practice, competency development and clinical decision making. Exemplars of advanced roles in minor injuries, emergency cardiology and psychiatric liaison have been included not only to illustrate real

Appendix 6: (*Continued*)

Year/Initiative/Report/Publication	Summary
	situations but also to assist those nurses and services interested in innovation in emergency nursing practice.
Profiles of Advanced Nurse/Midwife Practitioners and Clinical Nurse/Midwife Specialists (April)	This document showcases the work of a cross section of CNS/CMSs and ANP/AMPs, highlighting how the expansion of nursing and midwifery practice can meet patients'/clients' needs in flexible and innovative ways. Examples of care for people with heart failure, epilepsy, wounds, stroke, gastro-intestinal problems, diabetes, infections, autism, cervical cancer, mental health problems, pain and sexual health issues, in addition to end of life care, care of older people, neonates, occupational health and emergency care, are outlined. Common to all of the roles described here is how services have placed the patient/client at the centre and built service around their need, enhancing and integrating their journey through the health system.
Clinical Nurse Specialist/Clinical Midwife Specialist Resource Pack (Second Edition) (June)	The original version was developed in 2003 by the Nursing and Midwifery Planning Development Unit (NMPDU) in the former South-Eastern Health Board with funding from the National Council. It proved to be an important resource for clinical nurse and midwife specialists, many of

Appendix 6: (*Continued*)

Year/Initiative/Report/Publication	Summary
	whom were still adapting to their posts in a changing healthcare environment. The second edition of the *Clinical Nurse/Midwife Specialist Role Resource Pack* is the culmination of effective collaboration between national and regional bodies. This edition builds on the sound base provided by the first edition and incorporates the accumulated experience and expertise of both offices. A new first chapter outlines the developments in, and relevance to, the clinical career pathway that have taken place since the publication of the first edition in 2003. Elsewhere the references have been updated and text amended. A CD-ROM has been included which makes the templates and suggested activities more accessible. Finally, new case studies have been added with the aim of assisting the development of clinical specialist posts in intellectual disability, mental health, paediatrics and midwifery.
Clinical Supervision Discussion Paper (September)	The National Council supports nurses and midwives in developing and implementing new ways and approaches of continuing professional development (CPD) needs. This discussion paper aims to inform and stimulate debate and discussion about the role of clinical supervision in

Appendix 6: (*Continued*)

Year/Initiative/Report/Publication	Summary
	supporting CPD in the interests of improving quality patient care. Definitions and potential benefits of clinical supervision are outlined. Clinical supervision in Ireland is discussed in terms of its growing expansion and use in order to improve efficiency and effectiveness in the health service. Examples of clinical supervision from different perspectives in Ireland are outlined in order to offer insight for services planning to introduce clinical supervision.
NCNM Quarterly Review, Issues 29 and 30	The *NCNM Quarterly Review* continued to be used as a platform for the analysis and dissemination of information of relevance to the profession within the context of developments within the health services.

Appendix 7: Information on the Bologna Declaration

The Bologna Declaration is a joint declaration of the European ministers of education and was signed by thirty-one representatives of 29 EU member states and accession candidates in Bologna on 19 June 1999. It declares that by 2010 the following aims shall be reached:

1. A system of easily readable and comparable degrees shall be introduced, supported by the implementation of the Diploma Supplement.
2. Higher education course systems shall be based on two consecutive cycles: the undergraduate cycle, lasting three years, shall qualify students for employment; whereas the graduate cycle shall lead to masters' and/or doctorate degrees.
3. In order to ensure student mobility through the transferability of their achievements, a credit system similar to ECTS (European Credit Transfer and Accumulation System) shall be launched; credits shall also be obtainable in non-higher education contexts, such as life-long learning.
4. Student mobility and free movement shall be promoted.
5. European cooperation in quality assurance shall be established.
6. The European dimension shall be promoted in higher education through curricula, inter-institutional cooperation and mobility schemes for both students and teachers/researchers.

The ministers for education participating in the Bologna Process met in London in May 2007 and reaffirmed their commitment to the process. They stated that the aim is to replace the Bologna Process with the European Higher Education Area (EHEA) by 2010 and that by then there would be a single three year degree programme at undergraduate level throughout the area, with mutually recognised standards and accreditation. The purpose of this is to increase mobility and employability through the area.

References and Bibliography

Advisory Committee on Health Delivery and Human Resources (2003), *A Report on the Nursing Strategy for Canada*, Advisory Committee on Health Delivery and Human Resources, Canada, <www.scics.gc.ca/cinfo03/Nursing%20 Strategy.pdf>.

Advisory Committee on Health Human Resources (2000), *Nursing Strategy for Canada*, Advisory Committee on Health Human Resources, Canada, <http://www.hc-sc.gc.ca/hcs-sss/pubs/nurs-infirm/2000-nurs-infirm-strateg/index_e.html>.

Aguinaldo, J.P. (2004), `Rethinking the Validity of Qualitative Research from a Social Constructionist Perspective´, *The Qualitative Report*, 9(1): 127–136.

Aiken, L. (1995), `Transformation of the Nursing Workforce: The Shortage is in Properly Educated and Utilised Nurses´, *Nursing Outlook*, 43(5): 201–209.

Aiken, L., Smith, H. and Lake, E. (1994), `Lower Medicine Mortality among a set of Hospitals known for Good Nursing Care´, *Med Care*, 32(5): 771–787.

Aiken, L.H., Clarke, S.P., Cheung, R.B., Sloane, D.M. and Silber, J.H. (2003), `Educational Levels of Hospital Nurses and Surgical Patient Mortality´, *Journal of the American Medical Association*, 290(12): 1617–1623.

Aiken, L.H., Havens, D.S. and Sloane, D.M. (2000), `The Magnet Nursing Services Recognition Programme: A Comparison of Two Groups of Magnet Hospitals´, *American Journal of Nursing*, 100(3): 26–36.

An Bord Altranais (1994), *The Future of Nurse Education and Training*, Dublin: An Bord Altranais.

An Bord Altranais (1997), *Continuing Professional Education for Nurses in Ireland: A Framework*, Dublin: An Bord Altranais.

An Bord Altranais (2000a), *Scope of Nursing and Midwifery Practice Framework*, Dublin: An Bord Altranais.

An Bord Altranais (2000b), *Review of Scope of Practice for Nursing and Midwifery, Final Report*, Dublin: An Bord Altranais.

An Bord Altranais (2000c), *Requirements and Standards for Nurse Registration Education Programmes*, Dublin: An Bord Altranais.

An Bord Altranais (2000d), *Code of Professional Conduct for each Nurse and Midwife*, Dublin: An Bord Altranais.

An Bord Altranais (2001), *Guidelines for Midwives* (Third Edition), Dublin: An Bord Altranais.

An Bord Altranais (2005a), `Title Changes to the Division of the Register´, *An Bord Altranais News*, 17(1).

An Bord Altranais (2005b), *Annual Report 2005*, Dublin: An Bord Altranais.

An Bord Altranais (2005c), *Five Points Project*, <http://www.nursingboard.ie/en/spon-five_points.aspx>

An Bord Altranais (2007a), *Nurses Rules, 2007*, Dublin: An Bord Altranais.

An Bord Altranais (2007b), *Requirements and Standards for Education Programmes for Nurses and Midwives with Prescriptive Authority*, Dublin: An Bord Altranais.

An Bord Altranais (2007c), *Practice Standards for Nurses and Midwives with Prescriptive Authority*, Dublin: An Bord Altranais.

An Bord Altranais (2007d), *Decision-Making Framework for Nurse and Midwife Prescribing*, Dublin: An Bord Altranais.

An Bord Altranais (2007e), *Collaborative Practice Agreement for Nurses and Midwives with Prescriptive Authority*, Dublin: An Bord Altranais.

An Bord Altranais (2007f), *Annual Report 2006*, Dublin: An Bord Altranais.

An Bord Altranais and the National Council (2005), *Review of Nurses and Midwives in the Prescribing and Administration of Medicinal Products – Final Report*, Dublin: An Bord Altranais and the National Council for the Professional Development of Nursing and Midwifery.

Antrobus, A. and Kitson, A. (1999), `Nursing Leadership: Influencing and Shaping Health Policy and Nursing Practice´, *Journal of Advance Nursing*, 29(3): 746–753.

Arksey, H. and Knight, P. (1999), *Interviewing for Social Scientists: An Introductory Resource with Examples*, London: Sage Publications.

Australian Nursing and Midwifery Council (2004), *Nurse Practitioner Standards Project: Report to the Australian Nursing and Midwifery Council*, Dickson, ACT: Australian Nursing and Midwifery Council.

Axelsson, A., Kullén-Engström, A. and Edgren, L. (2000), `Management vs. Symbolic Leadership and Hospitals in Transition – A Swedish Example´, *Journal of Nursing Management*, 8(3): 167–173.

Balanda, K.P. and Wilde, J. (2001), *Inequalities in Mortality 1989–1998: A Report on All-Ireland Mortality Data*, Dublin: The Institute of Public Health in Ireland.

Barr, H. (2003), *Interprofessional Education: Today, Yesterday and Tomorrow – A Review*, commissioned by the Learning and Teaching Support Network for Health Sciences and Practice (LTSN) for the UK Centre for the Advancement of Interprofessional Education (CAIPE).

Barrington, R. (1987), *Health Medicine and Politics in Ireland 1900 to 1970*, Dublin: Institute of Public Administration.

Barron, S. and Kelly, C. (2006), *National Intellectual Disability Database Committee Annual Report 2006*, Dublin: Health Research Board.

Begley, C.M. (2002), '"Great Fleas have little Fleas": Irish Student Midwives´ Views of the Hierarchy in Midwifery', *Journal of Advanced Nursing*, 38(3): 310–317.

Begley, C.M., O'Boyle, C., Carroll, M. and Devane, D. (2007), 'Educating Advanced Midwife Practitioners: A Collaborative Venture', *Journal of Nursing Management*, 15: 574–584.

Benner, P. (1984), *From Novice to Expert: Excellence and Power in Clinical Nursing Practice*, Menlo Park, CA: Addison-Wesley Publishing Company.

Benner, P., Hooper-Kyriakidis, P. and Stannard, D. (1999), *Clinical Wisdom and Interventions in Critical Care: A Thinking-in-Action Approach*, Philadelphia, PA: Saunders.

Benz, C. and Newman, I. (1998), *Qualitative-Quantative Research Methodology: Exploring the Interactive Continuum*, Carbondale, IL: Southern Illinois University Press.

Berg, B.L. (1998), *Qualitative Research Methods for the Social Sciences*, Boston, MA: Allyn and Bacon.

Bower, F.L. (2000), 'Succession Planning: A Strategy for Taking Charge', *Nursing Leadership Forum*, 4(4): 110–113.

Bowles, A. and Bowles, N.B. (2000), 'A Comparative Study of Transformational Leadership in Nursing Development Units and Conventional Clinical Settings', *Journal of Nursing Management*, 8: 69–76.

Buresh, B. and Gordon, S. (2000), *From Silence to Voice: What Nurses Know and Must Communicate to the Public*, Ithaca, NY; London: ILR Press.

Campbell, M. (1987), 'Productivity in Canadian Nursing' in D. Colburn, G. D'Arcy and J. New (eds.) *Health in Canadian Society: Sociological Perspectives* (Second Edition), Toronto: McHenry & Whitesides.

Cardiovascular Health Strategy Group (1999), *Building Healthier Hearts: The Report of the Cardiovascular Health Strategy Group*, Dublin: The Stationery Office.

Carney, M. (1999), 'Leadership in Nursing: Where Do We Go from Here? The Ward Sisters Challenge for the Future', *Nursing Review*, 17(1/2): 13–18.

Carney, M. (2004), 'Middle Manager Involvement in Strategy Development in Not-for-Profit Organizations: The Director of Nursing Perspective – How Organizational Structure Impacts on the Role', *Journal of Nursing Management*, 12: 13–21.

Castledine, G. (1996), 'Clarifying and Defining Nursing Role Developments', *British Journal of Nursing*, 5(21): 1338.

Castledine, G. (2003a), 'Generalist and Specialist Nurses: Complementary or Conflicting Roles?' Unpublished paper delivered at Role Development Consensus Conference, Royal College of Physicians of Edinburgh, 17 November 2003.

Castledine, G. (2003b), 'Nurse Education and the NHS Must Integrate More', *British Journal of Nursing*, 12(17): 1055.

Castledine, G. (2004), 'Basic Nursing Principles Need to be Remembered', *British Journal of Nursing*, 13(6): 343.

Central Statistics Office (CSO) (2004a), *Population and Migration Estimates*, <http://www.cso.ie/statistics/documents/popmig. pdf>.

Central Statistics Office (CSO) (2004b), *Population and Labour Force Projections 2006–2036*, <http://www.cso.ie/releasespublications/po_lab_project_2006-2036.htm>.

Central Statistics Office (CSO) (2004c), *Irish Life Tables No. 14: 2001–2003*, <http://www.cso.ie/releasespublications/documents/births_d_m/current/irishlife.pdf>.

Central Statistics Office (CSO) (2004d), *Vital Statistics 3rd Quarter 2004*, <http://www.cso.ie/releasespublications/documents/vitalstats/2004/annualreport_2004.pdf>.

Central Statistics Office (CSO) (2006), *Census of the Population Statistics*, <http://www.cso.ie/census/>.

Central Statistics Office (CSO) (2007a), *Principal Causes of Death 1998–2006*, <http://www.cso.ie/statistics/principalcausesofdeath.htm>.

Central Statistics Office (CSO) (2007b), *Measuring Ireland's Progress 2006*, Dublin: The Stationery Office.

Chavasse, J. (2000), 'Nursing Education', in J. Robins (ed.), *Nursing and Midwifery in Ireland in the Twentieth Century*, Dublin: An Bord Altranais.

Commission of Enquiry on Mental Handicap (1965), *Report of the Commission of Enquiry on Mental Handicap*, Dublin: The Stationery Office.

Commission on Financial Management and Control Systems in the Health Service (2003), *Report of Commission on Financial Management and Control Systems in the Health Service (Brennan Report)*, Dublin: The Stationery Office.

Commission on Health Funding (1989), *Report of the Commission on Health Funding*, Dublin: The Stationery Office.

Commission on Nursing (1997), *Commission on Nursing Interim Report*, Dublin: The Stationery Office.

Commission on Nursing (1998), *Report of the Commission on Nursing: A Blueprint for the Future*, Dublin: The Stationery Office.

Commission on Patient Safety and Quality Assurance (2008), *Building a Culture of Patient Safety: Report of the Commission on Patient Safety and Quality Assurance*, Dublin: The Stationery Office.

Community Midwifery Service, National Maternity Hospital (2001), *The National Maternity Hospital Domino and Hospital*

Outreach Home Birth Service: Pilot Project Evaluation, Dublin: Women's Health Unit, Northern Area Health Board.

Condell, S. (1998), *Changes in the Professional Role of Nurses in Ireland: 1980–1997. A Report Prepared for the Commission on Nursing*, Dublin: The Stationery Office.

Condon, D. (2004), 'How to Attract Staff and Keep Them', *The World of Irish Nursing*, 12(1): 19–20.

Council of European Communities (1980), *Council Directive (80/155/EEC) Concerning the Coordination of Provisions laid down by Law, Regulation or Administrative Action Relating to the Taking up or Pursuit of the Activities of Midwives*, Brussels: Council of European Communities.

Cowen, B. (1998), Speech by the Minister for Health and Children, Mr Brian Cowen TD, on the publication of the *Report of the Commission on Nursing*, 16 September 1998, Dublin: Department of Health and Children.

Creswell, J.W. (1998), *Qualitative Inquiry and Research Design: Choosing Among Five Traditions*, London: Sage Publications.

Crossan, F. (2003), 'Strategic Management and Nurses: Building Foundations', *Journal of Nursing Management*, 11(5): 331–335.

DATHs Nursing Recruitment and Retention Group (2000), *DATHs Nursing Recruitment and Retention Group Report, 2000*, Dublin: Dublin Academic Teaching Hospitals.

Department of Health (1984), *The Psychiatric Services: Planning for the Future*, Dublin: The Stationery Office.

Department of Health (1986), *Health: The Wider Dimensions. A Consultative Statement on Policy*, Dublin: Department of Health and Children.

Department of Health (1988), *The Years Ahead: A Policy for the Elderly*, Dublin: The Stationery Office.

Department of Health (1994), *Shaping a Healthier Future: A Strategy for Effective Health Care in the 1990s*, Dublin: The Stationery Office.

Department of Health and Children (1997a), *Statement of Strategy*, Dublin: Department of Health and Children.

Department of Health and Children (1997b), *A Plan for Women's Health 1997 to 1999*, Dublin: Department of Health and Children.

Department of Health and Children (1998), *Strategy Statement 1998–2001: Working for Health and Well-Being*, Dublin: Department of Health and Children.

Department of Health and Children (1999a), *Children First: National Guidelines for the Protection and Welfare of Children*, Dublin: The Stationery Office.

Department of Health and Children (1999b), Statutory Instrument No. 376 of 1999, *National Council for the Professional Development of Nursing and Midwifery (Establishment Order, 1999)*, Dublin: The Stationery Office.

Department of Health and Children (2000), *The National Health Promotion Strategy 2000–2005*, Dublin: The Stationery Office.

Department of Health and Children (2001a), *Quality and Fairness: A Health System for You*, Dublin: The Stationery Office.

Department of Health and Children (2001b), *Primary Care: A New Direction*, Dublin: The Stationery Office.

Department of Health and Children (2001c), *Effective Utilisation of Professional Skills of Nurses and Midwives*, Dublin: Department of Health and Children.

Department of Health and Children (2002a), *The Health of our Children: Annual Report of the Chief Medical Officer*, Dublin: Department of Health and Children.

Department of Health and Children (2002b), *National Study of Turnover in Nursing and Midwifery*, Dublin: Department of Health and Children.

Department of Health and Children (2003a), *The Health Service Reform Programme*, Dublin: The Stationery Office.

Department of Health and Children (2003b), *Ireland's Changing Heart: Second Report on Implementation of the Cardiovascular Health Strategy*, Dublin: The Stationery Office.

Department of Health and Children (2003c), *Nurses' and Midwives' Understanding and Experiences of Empowerment in Ireland*, Dublin: Department of Health and Children, Nursing Policy Division.

Department of Health and Children (2003d), *A Research Strategy for Nursing and Midwifery in Ireland: Final Report*, Dublin: The Stationery Office.

Department of Health and Children (2003e), *Evaluation of the Irish Pilot Programme for the Education of the Healthcare Assistants*, Dublin: The Stationery Office.

Department of Health and Children (2003f), *Report of the National Task Force on Medical Staffing 2003: The Challenge for Nursing and Midwifery – A Discussion Paper*, Dublin: Department of Health and Children.

Department of Health and Children (2004a), *Health Information: A National Strategy*, Dublin: The Stationery Office.

Department of Health and Children (2004b), Statutory Instrument No. 494 of 2004, *European Communities (Organisation of Working Time) (Activities of Doctors in Training) Regulations 2004*, Dublin: The Stationery Office.

Department of Health and Children (2005a), the Health Service Reform Programme website: <http://www.healthreform.ie>.

Department of Health and Children (2005b), Statutory Instrument No. 132 of 2005, *Interim Health Information and Quality Authority (Establishment) Order, 2005*, Dublin: The Stationery Office.

Department of Health and Children (2007a), Statutory Instrument No. 200 of 2007, *Misuse of Drugs (Amendment) Regulations 2007*, Dublin: The Stationery Office.

Department of Health and Children (2007b), Statutory Instrument No. 201 of 2007, *Medicinal Products (Prescription and Control of Supply) (Amendment) Regulations 2007*, Dublin: The Stationery Office.

Department of Health and Children (2007c) *Health in Ireland: Key Trends 2007*, Dublin: Department of Health and Children.

Department of Health (Britain) (1989), *Working for Patients*, Cm 555, London: HMSO.

Department of Health (Britain) (1992), *Patients' Charter*, London: HMSO.

Department of Health (Britain) (1998), *A First Class Service: Quality in the New NHS*, Leeds: Department of Health.

Department of Health (Britain) (1999), *Making a Difference: Strengthening the Nursing, Midwifery and Health Visiting Contribution to Health and Health Care*, London: HMSO.

Department of Health (Britain) (2000), *The NHS Plan: A Plan for Investment, A Plan for Reform*, London: HMSO.

Department of Health (Britain) (2006), *Modernising Nursing Careers: Setting the Direction*, London: HMSO.

DHSSPS (Department of Health, Social Services and Public Safety, Northern Ireland) (1998), *Valuing Diversity… A Way Forward: A Strategy for Nursing, Midwifery and Health Visiting – 1998*, Belfast: DHSSPS.

DHSSPS (Department of Health, Social Services and Public Safety, Northern Ireland) (2003), *Valuing Diversity… A Way Forward: A Strategy for Nursing, Midwifery and Health Visiting - 1998. Summary of Achievements 1998–2003*, Belfast: DHSSPS.

DHSSPS (Department of Health, Social Services and Public Safety, Northern Ireland) (2004), *A Healthier Future: A Twenty-Year Vision for Health and Well-being in Northern Ireland*, Belfast: DHSSPS.

DHSSPS/DoHC (Department of Health, Social Services and Public Safety, Northern Ireland and Department of Health and Children, Dublin) (2001), *A Nursing Vision of Public Health: All Ireland Statement on Public Health and Nursing*, Belfast and Dublin: DHSSPS and Department of Health and Children.

DHSSPS/DoHC (Department of Health, Social Services and Public Safety, Northern Ireland and Department of Health and Children, Dublin) (2003), *From Vision to Action: Strengthening the Nursing Contribution to Public Health*, Belfast and Dublin: DHSSPS and Department of Health and Children.

DHSSPS/DoHC (Department of Health, Social Services and Public Safety, Northern Ireland and Department of Health and Children, Dublin) (2005), *Nursing for Public Health: Realising the Vision*, Belfast and Dublin: DHSSPS and Department of Health and Children.

Department of Health Western Australia (2003), *Guiding Framework for the Implementation of Nurse Practitioners in Western Australia*, Perth, W.A.: DHWA.

Department of the Taoiseach (1996), *Delivering Better Government: Second Report to the Government of the Coordinating Group of Secretaries – A Programme of Change for the Irish Civil Service*, Dublin: The Stationery Office.

Department of Tourism, Sport and Recreation (2001), *Building on Experience: National Drugs Strategy 2001–2008*, Dublin: The Stationery Office.

Downs, F. (1999), *Readings in Research Methodology*, Philadelphia, PA: Lippincott Williams & Wilkins.

Dublin Hospital Initiative Group (1991), *Reports* (three) *of the Dublin Hospital Initiative Group 1990–1991*, Dublin: The Stationery Office.

Duffy, K., Ferguson, C. and Watson, H. (2004), 'Data Collecting in Grounded Theory: Some Practical Issues', *Nurse Researcher*, 11(4): 67–79.

Dunham, J. and Klafehn, K. (1990), 'Transformational Leadership and the Nurse Executive', *Journal of Nursing Administration*, 20(4): 28–33.

Economic and Social Research Institute (ESRI) (2002), *Activity in Acute Public Hospitals in Ireland 1990–1999*, Dublin: ESRI.

Economic and Social Research Institute (ESRI) (2003), *Bed Occupancy Rates in Irish Health Care Institutions 2003*, Dublin: ESRI.

Economic and Social Research Institute (ESRI) (2008), *Medium Term Review 2008–2015*, Dublin: ESRI.

European Ministers of Education (1999), *European Higher Education Area – Joint Declaration of the European Ministers of Education*, Convened in Bologna on 19 June 1999, <ec.europa.eu/education/policies/educ/bologna/bologna.pdf>.

Expert Group on Mental Health Policy (2006), *A Vision for Change: Report of the Expert Group on Mental Health Policy*, Dublin: The Stationery Office.

Fahey, T., Russell, H. and Whelan, L.T. (2007), *Best of Times? The Social Impact of the Celtic Tiger*, Dublin: Institute of Public Administration.

FÁS (2005), *Health Care Skills Monitoring Report*, Dublin: FÁS.

Flynn, M. (1998), *Management in the Health Services: The Role of the Nurse – A Report Prepared for the Commission on Nursing*, Dublin: The Stationery Office.

Fradd, L. (2004), 'Political Leadership in Action', *Journal of Nursing Management*, 12(4): 242–245.

Frechtling, J. and Westat, L.S. (eds) (1997), 'User Friendly Handbook for Mixed Method Evaluations', *National Science Foundation*, <http://www.nsf.gov/pubs/1997/nsf97153/start.htm>.

Friel, S., Nic Gabhainn, S. and Kelleher, C. (1999), *The National Health and Lifestyle Surveys: Survey of Lifestyle Attitudes and Nutrition (SLAN) and the Irish Health Behaviour in School-Age Children (HBSC)*, Galway: Centre for Health Promotion Studies.

Friese, S. (2004), 'Software Overview', *Qualitative Research and Consulting*, Bissendorf, Germany, <http://www.quarc.de/software_overview_table.pdf>.

George, J. (1996), *Nursing Theories: The Base for Professional Nursing Practice* (Fourth Edition), Norwalk, CT: Appleton and Lang.

Government of Ireland (1919), *The Nurses Registration Act 1919*, Dublin: The Stationery Office.

Government of Ireland (1950), *Nurses Act, 1950*, Dublin: The Stationery Office.

Government of Ireland (1961), *Nurses Act, 1961*, Dublin: The Stationery Office.

Government of Ireland (1970), *Health Act, 1970*, Dublin: The Stationery Office.

Government of Ireland (1985), *Nurses Act, 1985*, Dublin: The Stationery 0ffice.

Government of Ireland (1994), *Strategic Management Initiative*, Dublin: The Stationery Office.

Government of Ireland (1997a), *Public Services Management Act 1997*, Dublin: The Stationery Office.

Government of Ireland (1997b), *Freedom of Information Act 1997*, Dublin: The Stationery Office.

Government of Ireland (2001), *Mental Health Act 2001*, Dublin: The Stationery Office.

Government of Ireland (2004), *Health Act, 2004*, Dublin: The Stationery Office.

Government of Ireland (2007a), *Irish Medicines Board (Miscellaneous Provisions) Act 2006 (Commencement) Order 2007*, Dublin: The Stationery Office.

Government of Ireland (2007b), *Health Act 2007*, Dublin: The Stationery Office.

Government of Ireland Inter-Departmental Group (2000), *The National Children's Strategy: Our Children – Their Lives*, Dublin: The Stationery Office.

Great Britain (1990), *National Health Service and Community Care Act 1990: Elizabeth II. Chapter 19*, London: The Stationery Office.

Griffin, M. and Melby, V. (2006), 'Developing an Advanced Nurse Practitioner Service in Emergency Care: Attitudes of Doctors and Nurses', *Journal of Advanced Nursing*, 56(3): 292–301.

Griffiths, R. (1983), *NHS Management Inquiry (The Griffiths Report)*, London: Department of Health and Social Security.

Hanafin, S. (1997), 'The Role of the Irish Public Health Nurse: Manager, Clinician and Health Promoter', *Health Visitor*, 70(8): 295–297.

Hanafin, S., Houston, A.M. and Cowley, S. (2002), 'Vertical Equity in Service Provision: A Model for the Irish Public Health Nursing Service', *Journal of Advanced Nursing*, 39(1): 68–76.

Health Research Board (HRB) (2002), *Making Knowledge Work for Health: A Strategy for Health Research*, Dublin: Department of Health and Children.

Health Service Executive (HSE) (2005), *Reach Out: A National Strategy for Action on Suicide Prevention*, Dublin: Health Service Executive.

Health Service Executive (HSE) (2006a), *Leas Cross Review*, Dublin: Health Service Executive.

Health Service Executive (HSE) (2006b), *Transformation Programme 2007–2010*, Dublin: Health Service Executive.

Health Service Executive (HSE) (2006c), *Expert Advisory Groups*, Dublin: Health Service Executive.

Health Service Executive (HSE) (2006d), 'Message from the CEO', *Health Matters*, Summer, Dublin: Health Service Executive.

Health Service Executive (HSE) (2006e), *A Strategy for Practice Development*, Waterford: Health Service Executive South-East Nursing and Midwifery Planning and Development Unit.

Health Service Executive (HSE) (2007a), *Nursing and Midwifery Turnover Data Report for Year Ending 2005 for HSE Areas of Counties Dublin, Kildare and Wicklow*, Dublin: HSE Nursing and Midwifery Planning and Development Unit for the Counties of Dublin, Kildare and Wicklow.

Health Service Executive (HSE) (2007b), 'A Time of Unlimited Opportunity for Nursing and Midwifery', *Health Matters*, Autumn, Dublin: Health Service Executive.

Health Service Executive (HSE) (2007c), 'HSE Transformation Programme and PCCC Programme', *Health Matters*, Summer, Dublin: Health Service Executive.

Health Service Executive (HSE) (2007d), *The Introduction of Nurse and Midwife Prescribing in Ireland: An Overview*, Dublin: Health Service Executive.

Health Service Executive (HSE) (2007e), *A Literature Review of Post-Registration Nursing and Midwifery Education: An Interim Report*, Unpublished.

Health Service Executive (HSE) (2007f), *A Literature Review of Post-Registration Nursing and Midwifery Education: A Report Commissioned by the Post-Registration and Post-Graduate Nursing and Midwifery Education Review Group*, Unpublished.

Health Service Executive (HSE) (2007g), *eLearning Guru*, <https://elearning.hseland.ie/tohm/default.asp>.

Health Service Executive (HSE) (2007h), *Overview of Nursing Careers in Ireland*, <http://www.careersinhealthcare.ie/nursing/overview.asp#cnm1>.

Health Service Executive (HSE) (2008a), *Employment in the Public Health Service 1997–2006*, <http://www.hse.ie/eng/FactFile/FactFile_PDFs/Other_FactFile_PDFs/Employment_In_The_Health_Service_Health_In_Ireland_Report.pdf>.

Health Service Executive (HSE) (2008b), *Transformation Programme Staff Briefing July 2008: National Integration – Local Responsibility*, <http://www.hse.ie/eng/newsmedia/Transformation_Programme_Staff_Briefing_July_2008.pdf>.

Health Service Executive Employers Agency (2007), 'New Deadline for Implementation of the European Working Time Directive for NCHDs', *Health Service Executive Employers Agency Newsletter*, Summer, Dublin: Health Service Executive.

Henderson, V. (1961), *Basic Principles of Nursing Care*, London: International Council of Nurses.

Henderson, V. (1966), *The Nature of Nursing: A Definition and its Implications for Practice, Research, and Education*, New York, NY: Macmillan.

Hennessy, D.A., Rowland, H. and Buckton, K. (1993), 'The Corporate Role of the Nursing Director', *Journal of Nursing Management*, 1: 161–169.

Hennessy, D.A. and Gilligan, J.H. (1994), 'Identifying and Developing Tomorrow's Trust Nursing Directors', *Journal of Nursing Management*, 2: 37–45.

Interim Health Information and Quality Authority (2007), 'Interim Health Information and Quality Authority to Play Supporting Role in New Commission on Patient Safety and Quality Assurance', *Interim Health Information and Quality Authority News Update*, March.

Irish Times (2006), 'New Body to Monitor Health Spending', *Irish Times Health Supplement*, 19 September 2006.

Irish Times (2007a), 'Drumm Expands Plans for North-East Services', *Irish Times Health Supplement*, 31 July 2007.

Irish Times (2007b), 'HSE Seeks €500 Million Savings in New Plan', *Irish Times Health Supplement*, 20 March 2007.

Irish Times (2007c), 'Shared Online Patient Files are Saving Time, Money', *Irish Times Health Supplement*, 10 April 2007.

Irish Times (2007d), 'Bringing Care Back Home', *Irish Times Health Supplement*, 17 July 2007.

Irish Times (2007e), 'State to Review Value of Nursing Degree', *Irish Times Health Supplement*, 31 July 2007.

Irish Times (2007f), 'Two Major Dublin Hospitals Join Forces', *Irish Times Health Supplement*, 7 August 2007.

Irish Times (2007g), 'Cancer Specialist Condemns Diagnosis System', *Irish Times*, 8 August 2007.

Irish Times (2007h), 'Value-for-Money Review is Futile and Flawed', *Irish Times Health Supplement*, 14 August 2007.

Irish Times (2007i), 'There is Now a Real Concern for Patient Safety', *Irish Times Weekend Review*, 22 September 2007.

Irvine, D., Leatt, P., Evans, M. and Baker, R. (1999), 'Measurement of Staff Empowerment Within Health Service Organisations', *Journal of Nursing Measurement*, 7(1): 79–95.

Janesick, V.J. (2003), 'The Choreography of Qualitative Research Design: Minuets, Improvisation and Crystallization', in N.K. Denzin and Y. Lincoln (eds), *Strategies of Qualitative Inquiry* (Second Edition), London: Sage Publications.

Johnson, R.B. (1997), 'Examining the Validity Structure of Qualitative Research', *Education*, 118(2): 282–290.

Jones, M.L. (2005), 'Role Development and Effective Practice in Specialist and Advanced Practice Roles in Acute Hospital Settings: Systematic Review and Meta-Synthesis', *Journal of Advanced Nursing*, 49(2): 191–209.

Kanter, R.M. (1993), *Men and Women of the Corporation*, New York, NY: Basic Books.

Kelleher, A. and Musgrave, E. (2000), 'Sick Children's Nursing', in J. Robins (ed) *Nursing and Midwifery in Ireland in the Twentieth Century*, Dublin: An Bord Altranais.

Kelleher, C., Nic Gabhainn, S., Friel, S., Corrigan, H., Nolan, G., Sixsmith, J., Walsh, O. and Cooke, M. (2003), *The National Health and Lifestyle Surveys: Survey of Lifestyle Attitudes and Nutrition (SLAN) and the Irish Health Behaviour in School Age Children (HBSC)*, Galway: Centre for Health Promotion Studies.

Kelly, F., Kelly, C. and Craig, S. (2007), *Annual Report of the National Intellectual Disability Database Committee 2007*, Dublin: Health Research Board.

Kennedy, P. (2002), *Maternity Care in Ireland: A Woman-Centred Perspective*, Dublin: Liffey Press.

King's Fund (1996), *Leadership Programme*, London: King's Fund.

King's Fund (2006), *Grow Your Own: Creating the Conditions for Sustainable Workforce Development*, London: King's Fund.

Kitson, A. (1999), 'The Essence of Nursing', *Nursing Standard*, 13(23): 42–46.

Klakovich, M. (1995), 'Development and Psychometric Evaluation of the Reciprocal Empowerment Scale', *Journal of Nursing Measurement*, 3(2): 127–143.

Kuokkanen, L. and Leino-Kilpi, H. (2000), 'Power and Empowerment in Nursing: Three Theoretical Approaches', *Journal of Advanced Nursing*, 31(1): 235–241.

Kuokkanen, L. and Leino-Kilpi, H. (2001), 'The Qualities of an Empowered Nurse and the Factors Involved', *Journal of Nursing Management*, 9: 273–280.

Labour Court (1997), Recommendation No. LRC 15450, CD/97/48, Dublin: Labour Court.

Laing, R.D. (1971), *The Politics of the Family and Other Essays*, New York, NY: Pantheon.

Laschinger, H.K.S. (2001), 'Impact of Structural and Psychological Empowerment on Job Strain in Nursing Work Settings', *Journal of Nursing Administration*, 31(5): 260–272.

Laschinger, H.K.S., Finnegan, J., Shamian, J. and Casier, S. (2001), 'Organizational Trust and Empowerment in Restructured Healthcare Settings', *Journal of Nursing Administration*, 30(9): 413–425.

Laschinger, H.K.S., Wong, C., McMahon, L. and Kaufmann, C. (1999), 'Leader Behavior Impact on Staff Nurse Empowerment, Job Tension and Work Effectiveness', *Journal of Nursing Administration*, 29(5): 28–39.

Lavin, M.A., Ruebling, I., Banks, R., Block, L., Counte, M., Furman, G., Miller, P., Reese, C., Viehmann, V. and Holt, J. (2001), 'Interdisciplinary Professional Education: A Historical Review', *Advances in Health Science Education*, 6(1): 25–47.

Leahy-Warren, P. (1998), *Community Nursing – An International Perspective. A Report prepared for the Commission on Nursing*, Dublin: The Stationery Office.

Leahy-Warren, P. and Tyrrell, M.P. (1998), *Joint Appointments in Nursing: A Report Prepared for the Commission on Nursing*, Dublin: The Stationery Office.

Lincoln, Y.S. and Guba, E.G. (1985), *Naturalistic Inquiry*, Newbury Park, CA: Sage Publications.

Lincoln, Y.S. and Guba, E.G. (2003), 'Paradigmatic Controversies, Contradictions and Emerging Confluences', in N.K. Denzin and Y. Lincoln (eds), *The Landscape of Qualitative Research: Theories and Issues* (Second Edition), London: Sage Publications.

Locke, K. (2001), *Grounded Theory in Management Research*, London: Sage Publications.

Mac Lellan, K. (2007), 'Expanding Practice: Developments in Nursing and Career Pathways', *Nursing Management* (Harrow), 14(3): 28–34.

Mantzoukas, S. and Watkinson, S. (2007), 'Review of Advanced Nursing Practice: The International Literature and Developing the Generic Features', *Journal of Clinical Nursing*, 16(1): 28–37.

Marsden, J., Dolan, B. and Holt, L. (2003), 'Nurse Practitioner Practice and Deployment: Electronic Mail Delphi Study', *Journal of Advanced Nursing*, 43(6): 595–605.

Mason, J. (1996), *Qualitative Researching*, London: Sage Publications.

Maternity Services Review Group (2001), *Report of the Maternity Services Review Group*, Drogheda: North-Eastern Health Board.

Mathers, N., Fox, N. and Hunn, A. (1998), *Trent Focus for Research and Development in Primary Health Care: Using Interviews in a Research Project*, Trent: Trent Focus Group.

Maxwell, J.A. (1992), 'Understanding and Validity in Qualitative Research', *Harvard Education Review*, 62(3): 279–300.

McCarthy, G., Tyrrell, M.P. and Cronin, C. (2002), *National Study of Turnover in Nursing and Midwifery*, Dublin: Department of Health and Children.

McKenna, H.P., Keeney, S. and Bradley, M. (2004), 'Nurse Leadership within Primary Care: The Perceptions of Community Nurses, GPs, Policy Makers and Members of the Public', *Journal of Nursing Management*, 12: 169–76.

Medel-Anonuevo, C., Ohsako, T. and Mauch, V. (2001), *Revisiting Lifelong Learning for the 21st Century*, Hamburg: UNESCO Institute for Education.

Mid-Western Health Board, NMPDU, Mid-Western Region (2003), *An Explorative Study into the Expansion of Nursing and Midwifery Professional Roles in Response to the European Working Time Directive*, Limerick: Mid-Western Health Board.

Miles, M.B. and Huberman, A.M. (1994), *Qualitative Data Analysis: An Expanded Sourcebook*, London: Sage Publications.

Ministry of Public Works and Government (2003), *A Report on the Nursing Strategy for Canada*, Ottawa, Ontario: Health Canada.

Myers, M. (2000), 'Qualitative Research and the Generalisability Question: Standing Firm with Proteus', *The Qualitative Report*, 4(3/4): 34–41.

National Advisory Committee on Palliative Care (2001), *Report of the National Advisory Committee on Palliative Care*, Dublin: The Stationery Office.

National Assembly for Wales (1999), *Realising the Potential: A Strategic Framework for Nursing, Midwifery and Health Visiting in Wales into the 21st Century*, Cardiff: National Assembly for Wales.

National Council (National Council for the Professional Development of Nursing and Midwifery) (2001a), *Clinical Nurse/Midwife Specialists Intermediate Pathway*, Dublin: National Council.

National Council (National Council for the Professional Development of Nursing and Midwifery) (2001b), *Framework for the Establishment of Advanced Nurse Practitioner and Advanced Midwife Practitioner Posts*, Dublin: National Council.

National Council (National Council for the Professional Development of Nursing and Midwifery) (2001c), *Criteria and Processes for the Allocation of Additional Funding for Continuing Education by the National Council*, Dublin: National Council.

National Council (National Council for the Professional Development of Nursing and Midwifery) (2002), *Guidelines on the Development of Courses Preparing Nurses and Midwives as Clinical Nurse/Midwife Specialists and Advanced Nurse/Midwife Practitioners*, Dublin: National Council.

National Council (National Council for the Professional Development of Nursing and Midwifery) (2003a), *Agenda for the Future Professional Development of Nursing and Midwifery*, Dublin: National Council.

National Council (National Council for the Professional Development of Nursing and Midwifery) (2003b), *Guidelines for Portfolio Development for Nurses and Midwives*, Dublin: National Council.

National Council (National Council for the Professional Development of Nursing and Midwifery) (2003c), *Guidelines for Health Service Providers for the Selection of Nurses and Midwives who might Apply for Financial Support in Seeking Opportunities to Pursue Further Education*, Dublin: National Council.

National Council (National Council for the Professional Development of Nursing and Midwifery) (2003d), *Guidelines for Portfolio Development for Nurses and Midwives*, Dublin: National Council.

National Council (National Council for the Professional Development of Nursing and Midwifery) (2004a), *Framework for the Establishment of Clinical Nurse/Midwife Specialist Posts Intermediate Pathway* (Second Edition), Dublin: National Council.

National Council (National Council for the Professional Development of Nursing and Midwifery) (2004b), *Framework for the Establishment of Advanced Nurse Practitioner and Advanced Midwife Practitioner Posts* (Second Edition), Dublin: National Council.

National Council (National Council for the Professional Development of Nursing and Midwifery) (2004c), *An Evaluation of the Effectiveness of the Role of Clinical Nurse/Midwife Specialist in Ireland*, Dublin: National Council.

National Council (National Council for the Professional Development of Nursing and Midwifery) (2004d), *Report on the Continuing Professional Development of Staff Nurses and Midwives*, Dublin: National Council.

National Council (National Council for the Professional Development of Nursing and Midwifery) (2005a), *Agenda for the Future Professional Development of Public Health Nursing*, Dublin: National Council.

National Council (National Council for the Professional Development of Nursing and Midwifery) (2005b), *Clinical Nurse Specialist and Advanced Nurse Practitioner Roles in Emergency Departments: Position Paper*, Dublin: National Council.

National Council (National Council for the Professional Development of Nursing and Midwifery) (2005c), *Service Needs*

Analysis for Clinical Nurse/Midwife Specialists and Advanced Nurse/Midwife Practitioners, Dublin: National Council.

National Council (National Council for the Professional Development of Nursing and Midwifery) (2005d), *A Study to Identify Research Priorities for Nursing and Midwifery in Ireland*, Dublin: National Council.

National Council (National Council for the Professional Development of Nursing and Midwifery) (2005e), *A Preliminary Evaluation of the Role of the Advanced Nurse Practitioner*, Dublin: National Council.

National Council (National Council for the Professional Development of Nursing and Midwifery) (2005f), *An Evaluation of the Extent and Nature of Nurse-led/Midwife-led Services in Ireland*, Dublin: National Council.

National Council (National Council for the Professional Development of Nursing and Midwifery) (2005g), *The Development of Joint Appointments: A Framework for Irish Nursing and Midwifery*, Dublin: National Council.

National Council (National Council for the Professional Development of Nursing and Midwifery) (2006a), *Review of Achievements 2001 to 2006*, Dublin: National Council.

National Council (National Council for the Professional Development of Nursing and Midwifery) (2006b), *Clinical Nurse Specialist and Advanced Nurse Practitioner Roles in Intellectual Disability Nursing: Position Paper 2*, Dublin: National Council.

National Council (National Council for the Professional Development of Nursing and Midwifery) (2006c), *Report on the Baseline Survey of Research Activity in Irish Nursing and Midwifery*, Dublin: National Council.

National Council (National Council for the Professional Development of Nursing and Midwifery) (2006d), *Guidelines for Portfolio Development for Nurses and Midwives* (Second Edition), Dublin: National Council.

National Council (National Council for the Professional Development of Nursing and Midwifery) (2006e), *Measurement of Nursing and Midwifery Interventions: Guidance and Resource Pack*, Dublin: National Council.

National Council (National Council for the Professional Development of Nursing and Midwifery) (2006f), *Improving the Patient Journey: Understanding Integrated Care Pathways*, Dublin: National Council.

National Council (National Council for the Professional Development of Nursing and Midwifery) (2007a), CNS/CMS and ANP/AMP Statistics, <http://www.ncnm.ie/default.asp?V_DOC_ID=990> and <http://www.ncnm.ie/default.asp?V_DOC_ID=974>.

National Council (National Council for the Professional Development of Nursing and Midwifery) (2007b) *Framework for the Establishment of Clinical Nurse Specialist and Clinical Midwife Specialist Posts* (Third Edition), Dublin: National Council.

National Council (National Council for the Professional Development of Nursing and Midwifery) (2007c) *Framework for the Establishment of Advanced Nurse Practitioner and Advanced Midwife Practitioner Posts* (Third Edition), Dublin: National Council.

National Council (National Council for the Professional Development of Nursing and Midwifery) (2007d) *Clinical Nurse Specialist and Advanced Nurse Practitioner Roles in Older Persons Nursing: Position Paper 3*, Dublin: National Council.

National Council (National Council for the Professional Development of Nursing and Midwifery) (2007e), *Criteria and Processes for the Allocation of Additional Funding for Continuing Education by the National Council* (Second Edition), Dublin: National Council.

National Council (National Council for the Professional Development of Nursing and Midwifery) (2008a), *Annual Report and Accounts 2007* (draft), Dublin: National Council.

National Council (National Council for the Professional Development of Nursing and Midwifery) (2008b), *A Framework for the Establishment of Advanced Nurse Practitioner and Advanced Midwife Practitioner Posts* (Fourth Edition), Dublin: National Council.

National Council (National Council for the Professional Development of Nursing and Midwifery) (2008c), *Accreditation of Advanced Nurse Practitioners and Advanced Midwife Practitioners* (Fourth Edition), Dublin: National Council.

National Council (National Council for the Professional Development of Nursing and Midwifery) (2008d), *Enhanced Nursing Practice in Emergency Departments: Position Paper 4*, Dublin: National Council.

National Council (National Council for the Professional Development of Nursing and Midwifery) (2008e), *Profiles of Advanced Nurse/Midwife Practitioners and Clinical Nurse/Midwife Specialists*, Dublin: National Council.

National Council (National Council for the Professional Development of Nursing and Midwifery) (2008f), *Clinical Supervision Discussion Paper*, Dublin: National Council.

National Council (National Council for the Professional Development of Nursing and Midwifery) and Health Service Executive (HSE), South (2008), *Clinical Nurse/Midwife Specialists Resource Pack* (Second Edition), Dublin: National Council and Health Service Executive, South.

National Task Force on Medical Staffing (2003), *Report of the National Task Force on Medical Staffing (Hanly Report)*, Dublin: Department of Health and Children.

National Task Force on Obesity (2005), *Obesity – The Policy Challenges: Report of the National Task Force on Obesity*, Dublin: Department of Health and Children.

National Task Force on Suicide (1998), *Report of the National Task Force on Suicide*, Dublin: The Stationery Office.

NEHB (North Eastern Health Board) (2001), *Report of the Maternity Services Review Group*, Drogheda: North Eastern Health Board.

Nelson Hagemaster, J. (1992), 'Life History: A Qualitative Method of Research', *Journal of Advanced Nursing*, 17(9): 1122–1128.

Neuman, B. (1995), *The Neuman Systems Model* (Third Edition), Norwalk, CT: Appleton and Lang.

Nightingale, F. (1860), *Notes on Nursing: What it Is, and What it is Not*, New York, NY: D. Appleton and Company.

Norman, I. and Cowley, S. (eds) (1999), *The Changing Nature of Nursing in a Managerial Age*, Oxford: Blackwell Science.

Nursing and Midwifery Resource Steering Group (2002), *The Nursing and Midwifery Resource: Final Report of the Steering Group – Towards Workforce Planning*, Dublin: The Stationery Office.

Nursing Council of New Zealand (2001), *The Nurse Practitioner*, Wellington: Nursing Council of New Zealand.

OECD (Organisation for Economic Co-operation and Development) (2007), *Health Data 2007: Statistics and Indicators for 30 Countries*, OECD, <http://www.oecd.org/health/healthdata>.

Office for Public Management (2001), *The Joint Appointments Guide: A Guide to Setting Up, Managing and Maintaining Joint Appointments for Health Improvements between Health Organisations and Local Government*, London: Office for Public Management.

O'Hara, T. (1998), 'Current Structure of the Irish Health Care System – Setting the Context', in A.L. Leahy and M.M. Wiley (eds), *The Irish Health System in the 21st Century*, Dublin: Oak Tree Press.

OHM (Office for Health Management) (1998), *Clinicians in Management – The Next Steps: Facilitating Management Development for the Health Services. A Report on a One Day Conference in Dublin Castle Launching a New Initiative to Promote Clinicians in Management*, Dublin: Office for Health Management.

OHM (Office for Health Management) (2000), *Report on Nursing Management Competencies*, Dublin: Office for Health Management.

OHM (Office for Health Management) (2003a), *Learning from the NHS in Change: A Study on the Management of Major Structural Change in the NHS*, Dublin: Office for Health Management.

OHM (Office for Health Management) (2003b), *Report on an Evaluation Study of the Leading an Empowered Organisation Programme (LEO) for Clinical Nurse Managers 1*, Dublin: Office for Health Management.

OHM (Office for Health Management) (2003c), *Report on the Diagnostic Exercise for Directors of Nursing/Equivalent Nursing Management Grades*, Dublin: Office for Health Management.

OHM (Office for Health Management) (2003d), *Clinicians in Management: Charter of Rights and Responsibilities of Consultants,*

Clinical Directors and Senior Hospital Managers within the Acute Hospital Setting, Dublin: Office for Health Management.

OHM (Office for Health Management) (2004a), *The Management Competency User Pack for Nurse and Midwife Managers*, Dublin: Office for Health Management.

OHM (Office for Health Management) (2004b), 'Leadership Development Programme Past Participants – Where are they Now?', *Office for Health Management Newsletter*, Issue 5.

Orb, A., Eisenhauer, L. and Wynaden, D. (2001), 'Ethics in Qualitative Research', *Journal of Nursing Scholarship*, 33(1): 93–96.

Orem, D.E. (1985), *Nursing: Concepts of Practice* (Third Edition), New York, NY: McGraw Hill.

O'Shea, Y. (1995) *Resource Management and the Clinical Directorate Model: Implications for St. James's Hospital, Dublin*, Unpublished M.Sc. Econ. Dissertation, University of Dublin, Trinity College.

Paediatric Nurse Education Review Group (2000), *Report of the Paediatric Nurse Education Review Group*, Dublin: Department of Health and Children, Nursing Policy Division.

PA Knowledge Ltd. (2007), *Acute Hospital Bed Review: A Review of Acute Hospital Bed Use in Hospitals in the Republic of Ireland with an Emergency Department*, London: PA Consulting Group.

Pan-Canadian Steering Committee (2005), *Building the Future: An Integrated Strategy for Nursing Human Resources in Canada – Phase I Final Report*, <http://www.buildingthefuture.ca>.

Prospectus Strategy Consultants (2003), *Audit of Structures and Functions in the Health System, 2003 (Prospectus Report)*, Dublin: The Stationery Office.

Qualis Research Associates (2001), *The Ethnograph v5.08 – eManual*, London: Qualis Research Associates.

Richardson, L. (1994), 'Writing: A Method of Inquiry', in N.K. Denzin and Y.S. Lincoln (eds) *Handbook of Qualitative Research*, Thousand Oaks, CA: Sage.

Robins, J. (2000), 'Bord Altranais 1950–1970', in J. Robins (ed), *Nursing and Midwifery in Ireland in the Twentieth Century*, Dublin: An Bord Altranais.

Robson, C. (2002), *Real World Research: A Resource for Social Scientists and Practitioner-Researchers,* London: Blackwell Publishing.

Rogers, C. (1976), *Introduction to Nursing: An Adaptation Model,* New York, NY: Prentice Hall.

Roper, N., Logan, W.W. and Tierney, A.J. (2000), *The Roper-Logan-Tierney Model of Nursing: Based on Activities of Living,* Edinburgh: Elsevier Health Sciences.

Savage, E.B. (1998), *An Examination of the Changes in the Professional Role of the Nurse Outside Ireland: 1980–1997. A Report Prepared for the Commission on Nursing,* Dublin: The Stationery Office.

Scanlan, M. (2006), 'The Policy Role of the Department of Health and Children within the Irish Health Services', National Council Annual Conference, 15 November 2006, Speech by Michael Scanlan, Secretary General, Department of Health and Children.

Scoble, K. and Russell, G. (2003), 'Vision 2020, Part 1: Profile of the Future Nurse Leader', *Journal of Nursing Administration,* 33(6): 324–330.

Scott, P.A., Hayes, E. and MacNeela, P. (2006), *An Exploration of the Core Nursing Elements of Care Provided by Registered General Nurses within the Community Setting,* Dublin: Dublin City University.

Scottish Executive Health Department (2001), *Caring for Scotland: The Strategy for Nursing and Midwifery in Scotland,* Edinburgh: Scottish Executive.

Sheridan, A. (2000), 'Psychiatric Nursing', in J. Robins (ed), *Nursing and Midwifery in Ireland in the Twentieth Century,* Dublin: An Bord Altranais.

Singleton, Jr., R.A. and Straits, B.C. (1999), *Approaches to Social Research,* New York, NY: Oxford University Press.

SKILL Project, <http://www.skillproject.ie>.

Sofarelli, D. (1998), 'The Need for Nursing Leadership in Uncertain Times', *Journal of Nursing Management,* 6(4): 201–207.

South West Thames Regional Authority (1992), *A Competency Framework for Trust Nursing Directors,* London: South West Thames Regional Health Authority.

St. James's Hospital (1996), *Tender for Establishment and Provision of Cardiac Surgery Services at St. James's Hospital*, Dublin: St. James's Hospital.

Stake, R.E. (2003), 'Case Studies', in N.K. Denzin and Y. Lincoln (eds), *Strategies of Qualitative Inquiry* (Second Edition), London: Sage Publications.

Storey, L. (2001), 'The Concept of Competence', *Assessment of Competence Conference Proceedings*, Dublin: An Bord Altranais.

Surridge, H. (2007), *Qualitative Research and Critical Appraisal*, Southampton, North-West Hampshire Research and Development Support Unit, 18 January 2007, Southampton General Hospital, <http://www.rdsu.soton.ac.uk/courses/F2-Trainees/F2%20Qual%20Crit%20Appr%202007.pdf>.

Taylor, C. (2005), *What Packages are Available?*, School of Human and Health Sciences, University of Huddersfield, England, <http://onlineqda.hud.ac.uk/Which_software/what_packages_are_available/index.php>.

Taylor, C. (2006), *Online QDA*, School of Human and Health Sciences, University of Huddersfield, England, <http://onlineqda.hud.ac.uk/glossary.php#s>.

Teamwork Management Services Ltd. (2006), *Health Service Executive: Improving Safety and Achieving Better Standards - An Action Plan for Health Service in the North-East*, Bolton: Teamwork Services Management Ltd.

TIGER (Technology Informatics Guiding Education Reform) (2007), *The TIGER Initiative – Evidence and Informatics Transforming Nursing: 3-Year Action Steps Towards a 10-Year Vision*, <https://www.tigersummit.com/uploads/TIGERInitiative_Report2007_bw.pdf>.

Titchen, A. (1998), *Professional Craft Knowledge in Patient-Centred Nursing and the Facilitation of its Development*, Unpublished D.Phil. Thesis, Department of Education Studies, University of Oxford.

Treacy, M.P. and Hyde, A. (2003), 'Developments in Nursing in Ireland: The Emergence of a Disciplinary Discourse', *Journal of Professional Nursing*, 19(2): 91–98.

Tutty, L.M., Rothery, M. and Grinnell, Jr., R.M. (1996), *Qualitative Research for Social Workers*, Boston, MA: Allyn and Bacon.

Tyrrell, M.P. (1998), *Developments in Pre-Registration Nursing Education – An International Perspective. A Report Prepared for the Commission on Nursing*, Dublin: The Stationery Office.

University College Dublin (2007), Information on Post of Professor of Clinical Nursing (Acute Care Nursing) and Professor of Clinical Nursing (Palliative Nursing), <https://www.ucd.ie>.

Upenieks, V. (2003), 'Nurse Leaders' Perceptions of What Comprises Successful Leadership in Today's Acute Inpatient Environment', *Nursing Administration Quarterly*, 27(2): 140–152.

Weitzman, E. and Miles, M.B. (1995), *Computer Programmes for Qualitative Data Analysis: A Software Source Book*, Boston, MA: University of Massachusetts.

West, E., Barron, D.N., Dowsett, J. and Newton, J.N. (1999), 'Hierarchies and Cliques in the Social Networks of Health Care Professionals: Implications for the Design of Dissemination Strategies', *Social Science and Medicine*, 48(5): 633–646.

West, E. and Rafferty, A.M. (2004), *The Future Nurse: Evidence of the Impact of Registered Nurses*, York: University of York.

Working Group on the Effective Utilisation of Professional Skills of Nurses and Midwives (2001), *Report of the Working Group on the Effective Utilisation of Professional Skills of Nurses and Midwives*, Dublin: Department of Health and Children.

Working Party on General Nursing (1980), *Report of the Working Party on General Nursing*, Dublin: The Stationery Office.

WHO (World Health Organisation) (1981), *Global Strategy for Health for All by the Year 2000*, Geneva: WHO.

WHO (World Health Organisation) (1988), *Learning Together to Work Together for Health*, Geneva: WHO.

WHO (World Health Organisation) (1993), *Nursing in Action: Strengthening Nursing and Midwifery to Support Health for All*, Copenhagen: WHO Regional Office.

WHO (World Health Organisation) (1994), *Nursing Beyond the Year 2000: Report of a WHO Study Group*, Geneva: WHO.

WHO (1996), *Nursing Practice: Report of a WHO Expert Committee*, Geneva: WHO.

WHO (World Health Organisation) (1997), *A Strategy for Nursing and Midwifery Development in the Eastern Mediterranean Region*, Alexandria: WHO Regional Office for the Eastern Mediterranean.

WHO (World Health Organisation) (1999), *Nurses and Midwives for Health: A WHO European Strategy for Nursing and Midwifery Education*, Copenhagen: WHO Regional Office.

WHO (World Health Organisation) (2001), *The Ideal Attributes of Chief Nurses in Europe: A Delphi Study for WHO Europe*, Copenhagen: WHO Regional Office.

WHO (World Health Organisation) (2002), *Nursing Midwifery Services: Strategic Directions 2002–2008*, Geneva: WHO.

WHO (World Health Organisation) (2003), *National Strategy and Plan of Action for Nursing and Midwifery Development in Iraq 2003–2008*, Alexandria: WHO Eastern Mediterranean Regional Office.

WHO (World Health Organisation) (2004), *Health for All Database*, Copenhagen: WHO Regional Office.

WHO Expert Committee on Nursing Practice (1996), *Nursing Practice: Report of a WHO Expert Committee*, Geneva: WHO.

Zwarenstein, M., Atkins, J., Barr, H., Hammick, M., Koppel, I. and Reeves, S. (1999), 'A Systematic Review of Interprofessional Education', *Journal of Interprofessional Care*, 13(4): 417–424.

Index